WORKBOOK FOR DIAGNOSTIC MEDICAL SONOGRAPHY

A Guide to Clinical Practice, Obstetrics and Gynecology

FIFTH EDITION

WORKBOOK FOR DIAGNOSTIC MEDICAL SONOGRAPHY

A Guide to Clinical Practice, Obstetrics and Gynecology

FIFTH EDITION

Barbara Hall-Terracciano, BS, RDMS
(OB)(AB)(BR), RT(R)
Sonographer
St. George, Utah

Susan R. Stephenson, MS, MAEd, RDMS, RVT
Siemens Medical Solutions USA, Inc.
Pagosa Springs, Colorada

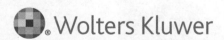. Wolters Kluwer

Philadelphia • Baltimore • New York • London
Buenos Aires • Hong Kong • Sydney • Tokyo

Acquisitions Editor: Nicole Dernoski
Development Editor: Eric McDermott
Editorial Coordinator: Oliver Raj
Marketing Manager: Kirstin Watrud
Production Project Manager: Frances M. Gunning
Manager, Graphic Arts & Design: Stephen Druding
Manufacturing Coordinator: Beth Welsh
Prepress Vendor: S4Carlisle Publishing Services

Fifth edition

9 8 7 6 5 4 3 2 1

Printed in Mexico

Library of Congress Cataloging-in-Publication Data

ISBN-13: 978-1-975177-02-7

ISBN-10: 1-975177-02-9

Cataloging in Publication data available on request from publisher.

shop.lww.com

CONTENTS

PART ONE

INTRODUCTION

CHAPTER 1

Orientation and Labeling in Obstetric and Gynecologic Imaging

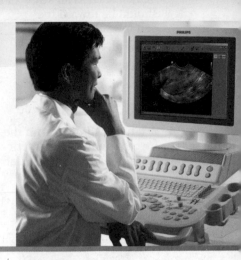

REVIEW OF GLOSSARY TERMS

Matching

Match the key terms with their definitions.

KEY TERMS

1. ____ Sims position

2. ____ fetal lie

3. ____ caudal

4. ____ morphology

5. ____ fetal presentation

6. ____ ventral

7. ____ cranial

8. ____ dorsal

9. ____ anatomic position

DEFINITION

a. Position of the fetus in utero
b. Left lateral decubitus position with the knees and thighs toward the chest
c. Toward the head or cranium
d. Body in the erect position with the palms forward and feet pointed forward
e. Form, structure, and location of organs
f. Toward the back or spine
g. Term used to describe which portion of the fetus will deliver first
h. Toward the belly or front
i. Toward the feet or tail end

CHAPTER REVIEW

Multiple Choice

Complete each question by circling the best answer.

1. The sagittal scan plane refers to a(n):
   a. vertical plane that divides the maternal or fetal body into superior and inferior sections
   b. axial views of the fetus or fetal patient
   c. vertical plane dividing the fetal or female body into right or left sections
   d. horizontal plane dividing the fetus or maternal patient into inferior and superior sections

2. The _____ view divides the patient body into anterior and posterior planes.
   a. transverse
   b. ventral
   c. lateral
   d. coronal

3. A transabdominal transducer provides a position indicator (i.e., notch, groove) comparable to an image marker such as an arrow or dot. The position indicator should be toward the _____ for longitudinal imaging and toward the patient's _____ in transverse imaging.
    a. head, left
    b. feet, left
    c. head, right
    d. feet, left

4. A fetus positioned with the cranium in the superior uterus, rump in the inferior uterus, and spine at the maternal right uterus is labeled:
    a. breech, left lateral
    b. vertex, left lateral
    c. breech, right lateral
    d. vertex, right lateral

5. Choose the position that is the same as a cephalic presentation.
    a. Frank breech
    b. Oblique
    c. Transverse
    d. Vertex

6. Minimal documentation on a technical impression worksheet should include:
    a. specific examination requested, patient address, relevant clinical information
    b. classification of disease identification code, physician contact information, technical impression
    c. examination date, patient name and identifiers, specific examination requested
    d. patient name and identifiers, patient height and weight, name of the patient's clinician and contact information

7. Select the inappropriate statement for a sonographer's technical impression.
    a. Ruptured ectopic pregnancy
    b. Retroflexed uterus
    c. Posterior cul-de-sac free fluid, 3.3 × 4.1 × 2.1 cm
    d. Heterogeneous right ovary with a 2 × 4 mm echogenic shadowing focus

8. Ipsilateral means:
    a. located or affecting the opposite side of the body
    b. closer to the attachment of an extremity to the trunk
    c. located or affecting the same side of the body
    d. toward the body surface or externally located

9. The aorta, inferior vena cava, and iliac vessels lie _____ to the female reproductive organs.
    a. deep
    b. rostral
    c. proximal
    d. contralateral

10. Select the incorrect gynecologic abbreviation:
    a. AF anteflexed
    b. FHR fundal height requirement
    c. OV ovary
    d. CX cervix

Fill-in-the-Blank

1. A endovaginal sagittal anteflexed or anteverted uterus image requires the transducer orientation marker to be placed at _____ o'clock.

2. The LPO position needs a patient to lie on the _____ posterior surface with a _____ anterior surface.

3. In obstetrics, RPOC means _____.

4. The _____ portion of the fallopian tube attaches onto the lateral uterus.

5. The term _____ indicates that the fetal buttocks are toward the cervix.

6. The term _____ indicates that the fetal cranium is positioned toward the cervix.

7. If the uterus does not lie in a true longitudinal or transverse position, it can be identified by _____, _____, or _____ the transducer to align it into an identifiable plane.

8. The abdominal wall is _____ to the uterus.

9. TAH means _____.

10. To direct fetal weight from the maternal great vessels use the _____ position and _____ position.

11. LGA means _____.

12. To identify cranial anatomy in late pregnancy when the transabdominal approach is not adequate, use either a _____ or _____ approach.

Short Answer

1. State pertinent clinical information that should be included in a sonographer's technical impression.

2. State the common interchangeable terms to describe the long axis of the uterus.

3. Explain the correct direction to rotate the TA or EV transducer to obtain a transverse image.

IMAGE EVALUATION/PATHOLOGY

Answer the following questions.

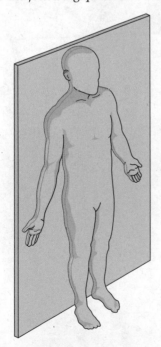 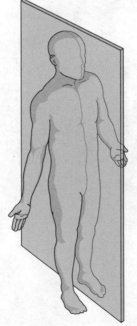 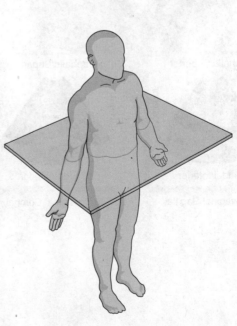

1. List the three common anatomic scan planes.

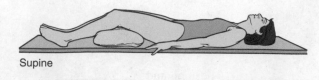

Supine

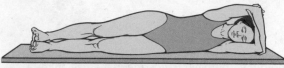

Lateral

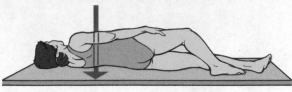

LPO

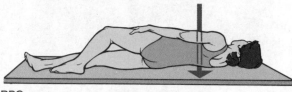

RPO

2. Name the patient positions used for transabdominal ultrasound scanning.

3. The apex of a transvaginal/endovaginal image corresponds to what part of the anatomy?

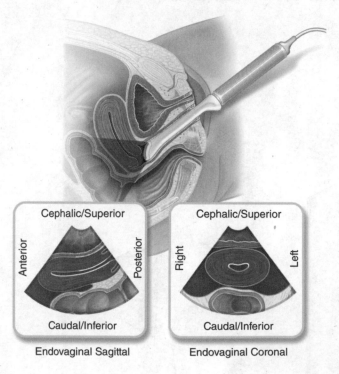

Endovaginal Sagittal   Endovaginal Coronal

Sonographic Image Optimization

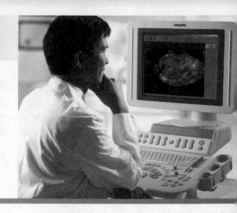

REVIEW OF GLOSSARY TERMS

Matching

Match the key terms with their definitions.

KEY TERMS

1. _____ temporal resolution

2. _____ qualitative

3. _____ lateral resolution

4. _____ spatial resolution

5. _____ cine-loop

6. _____ image resolution

7. _____ pixel

8. _____ region of interest

9. _____ color Doppler

10. _____ pulse repetition frequency (PRF)

11. _____ directional color power angio/directional power Doppler

12. _____ color power Doppler/power Doppler

13. _____ axial resolution

14. _____ quantitative

DEFINITION

a. Ability of the ultrasound system to display echoes as separate structures parallel to the transmitted beam

b. Series of 2D images providing a method to display movement (i.e., fetal heart)

c. Doppler data conversion into a nondirectional amplitude color overlay on the grayscale image

d. Doppler data conversion into a directional velocity color overlay on the grayscale image

e. Combination of directional color Doppler and nondirectional amplitude color Doppler modes

f. General term encompassing axial, lateral, spatial, contrast, and temporal resolution

g. Ability of the ultrasound system to display echoes as separate structures perpendicular to transmitted beam

h. One area, corresponding to the X and Y axis, of the 2D image

i. Number of cycles (frequency) of pulses per second

j. Numerical measurement

k. Description of quality of components without a numerical component

l. Area of data acquisition for color Doppler information

m. Ability of the ultrasound system to display echoes as separate structures that lie close together

n. Ability of the ultrasound system to display events occurring at different times (i.e., systole and diastole of the fetal heart)

CHAPTER REVIEW

Multiple Choice

Complete each question by circling the best answer.

1. Overall gain adjusts or amplifies the _____ of all the pixels on the system monitor.
   a. resolution
   b. brightness
   c. alphanumeric image information
   d. noise

2. As sound travels through tissue, there is a waveform amplitude _____ because of attenuation.
   a. scattering
   b. reflection
   c. reduction
   d. increase

3. TGC allows the adjustment of image by changing areas to:
   a. darker or brighter
   b. enlarge
   c. deeper visualization
   d. the near field

4. A single focal zone carat should be positioned:
   a. 1 cm superior to the central image
   b. at the lateral margin of the acquired structure
   c. 1 cm inferior to the desired anatomy
   d. at or just deep to the imaged structure

5. The best B-mode image uses:
   a. the lowest frequency that provides an adequate amount of penetration
   b. high resolution with a high frame rate
   c. the highest frequency that provides an adequate amount of penetration
   d. low frequency without aliasing

6. A higher dynamic range is best utilized with:
   a. the uterus
   b. ovarian varicosities
   c. fetal heart imaging
   d. the aorta

7. Narrowing sector width _____ frame rate.
   a. heightens
   b. widens
   c. decreases
   d. increases

8. Low persistence improves resolution of:
   a. ovarian masses
   b. the fetal heart
   c. breast masses
   d. uterine masses

9. The maps feature adjusts _____ of the grays in an image.
   a. brightness
   b. the number
   c. the size
   d. the shades

10. Which is not an indicator of thermal index?
    a. TIB
    b. TIC
    c. TIS
    d. TIA

11. Tissue harmonic imaging offers improved image by decreasing all except:
    a. side lobes
    b. reverberation
    c. speckle
    d. contrast

12. This feature uses multiple, averaged transmit beams at different angles and frequencies to increase image detail.
    a. Persistence
    b. FOV
    c. Compound imaging
    d. Maps

13. Sweep Speed adjusts the M-mode scrolling speed or:
    a. time
    b. pattern
    c. rhythm
    d. movement

14. Turbulent flow patterns are often associated with:
    a. normal pathology
    b. red coloring
    c. pathologies
    d. blue coloring

15. The optimal angle to sample with color flow is:
    a. 20 to 45 degrees
    b. 30 to 60 degrees
    c. 45 to 75 degrees
    d. 60 to 90 degrees

16. On a color bar indicator, the black area represents:
    a. turbulent flow
    b. range of flow velocities displayed above and below the baseline
    c. flow toward the transducer
    d. flow away from the transducer

17. What will aid in detecting slow vascular flow?
    a. Pressing "maps" control
    b. Decreasing persistence
    c. Increasing persistence
    d. Decreasing color priority

18. This type of artifact occurs when a structure is a strong reflector, such as fetal bony structures, or when a tissue reflects most or all of the transmitted beam.
    a. Posterior acoustic shadowing
    b. Posterior acoustic enhancement
    c. Reverberation
    d. Refraction

19. Movement of the transducer or targeted anatomy results in an artifact called:
    a. blooming
    b. color bleed
    c. color reversal
    d. color flash

20. Evaluation of a cystic structure results in the creation of an area deep into the targeted anatomy appearing:
    a. brighter than the adjacent tissue
    b. similar to the adjacent tissue
    c. with random noise
    d. darker than the adjacent tissue

Fill-in-the-Blank

1. "Slide pots" is another name for _____.

2. The control _____ is used when the overall appearance of the image is too bright or too dark.

3. Dynamic range or DR is simply the range of _____ displayed in the B-mode image.

4. Adding _____ or _____ to an image has the potential to increase structure visualization over black and white coloring.

5. Increasing persistence _____ the frame rate.

6. The mechanical index is an indicator of the _____ to tissue with the passing wave.

7. The M-mode or motion mode tracings provide a graphic display of structures in relation to _____.

8. If color appears outside of the vessel when using color Doppler gain, it indicates a _____ gain level.

9. Optimally, the ROI should be no larger than necessary because of the _____ frame rates often associated with a larger color box.

10. From a frame rate perspective, it is better to have a _____ ROI than a _____ ROI.

11. Changing the "Smooth" function adjusts the _____ averaging for flow between color frames.

12. The _____ selection reverses the color display.

13. Power Doppler is an alternate method for assessing _____-flow velocities.

14. The _____ function reduces the amount of noise and clutter by suppressing the lower-level signals that are the result of tissue and vessel wall motion.

15. The first step in obtaining a quality 3D data set is the optimization of the _____ image.

16. Extra beams, located adjacent to the central beam, called _____ create echoes in an incorrect location.

17. _____-mode provides a graphic display of motion in the fetal heart.

18. An image produced with misregistration of sound waves occurs when a structure lies between the transducer and a curved or with an angled strong reflector. It is called _____ or _____.

19. Color power Doppler uses amplitude to create a color _____ of blood flow.

20. The reduction of Doppler aliasing is through adjustment of the _____ or baseline.

Short Answer

1. List the types of Doppler modes.

2. Explain the 2D control: Res/Speed or Res/Pen, overall gain, and depth.

3. What is the difference between mirror image and grating lobe artifact?

IMAGE EVALUATION/PATHOLOGY

Answer the following questions.

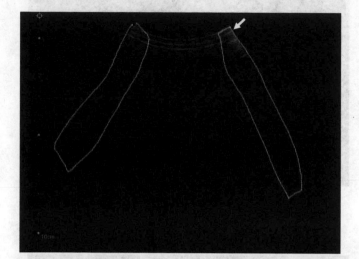

1. Explain what the arrow is directed at.

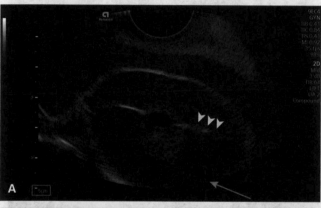

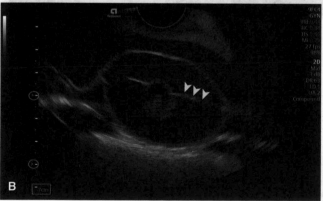

2. Describe the image differences. Take note of depth.

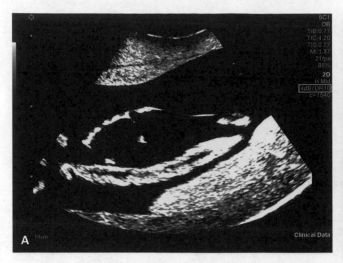 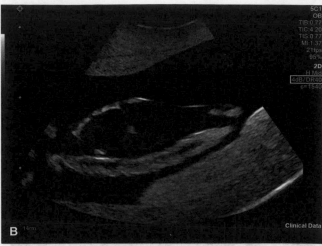

3. What is the dB and DR of the two images? Explain which is most diagnostic and why?

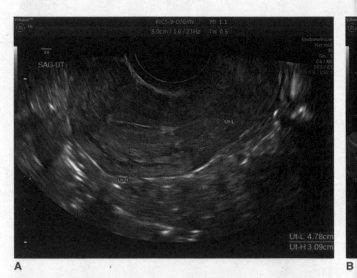 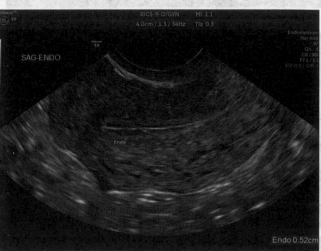

4. Discuss the image differences.

5. Name the artifact in the image.

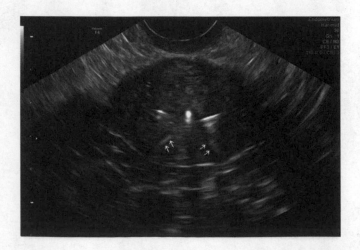

CHAPTER 3

Principles of Scanning Technique in Gynecologic Ultrasound

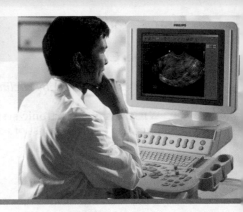

REVIEW OF GLOSSARY TERMS

Matching

Match the key terms with their definitions.

KEY TERMS

1. _____ fundus

2. _____ transabdominal

3. _____ electronic medical record (EMR)

4. _____ picture archiving and communication system (PACS)

5. _____ transvaginal/endovaginal

6. _____ scanning protocol

7. _____ bioeffects

8. _____ perivascular

9. _____ ascites

10. _____ transducer footprint

11. _____ adnexa

12. _____ modality worklist (MWL)

13. _____ lithotomy position

14. _____ endocavity

15. _____ radiology information system (RIS)

16. _____ nongravid

17. _____ hospital information system (HIS)

DEFINITION

a. Area around an organ
b. Fluid within the abdominal or pelvic cavity
c. Inside a cavity such as the abdomen or pelvis
d. Electronic database containing all the patient information
e. Biophysical results of the interaction of sound waves and tissue
f. Nonpregnant
g. Paper-based or computerized system designed to manage hospital data, such as billing and patient records
h. Position of the patient with the feet in stirrups often used during delivery
i. Imaging through the abdomen
j. Top portion of the uterus
k. Around the vessels
l. Database that stores radiologic images
m. Within the vagina
n. List of images required for a complete examination
o. Electronic list of patients entered into a modality, such as ultrasound, which helps reduce data entry errors
p. Area of the transducer that comes in contact with the patient and emits ultrasound
q. Physical or electronic system designed to manage radiology data, such as billing, reports, and images

CHAPTER REVIEW

Multiple Choice

Complete each question by circling the best answer.

1. What hospital electronic system would a sonographer use to locate a list of patients on the ultrasound machine?
   a. HIS
   b. RIS
   c. MWL
   d. EMR

2. Necessary clinical information for a pelvic sonographic examination and report may include:
   a. surgical history, patient age, LMP, hCG levels, prior delivery dates, gravidity, parity
   b. prior delivery dates, patient age, surgical history, gravidity, history of pelvic procedures
   c. LMP, symptoms, history of pelvic procedures, patient age, hCG levels, accession number
   d. parity, gravidity, symptoms, pelvic history to include pelvic procedures, surgical history

3. Parity is:
   a. the number of pregnancies a patient has had
   b. the total number of spontaneous and induced abortions a patient has had
   c. the number of pregnancies a patient carried to term
   d. the total number of pregnancies a patient has had

4. A G4P3A1T3 female is explained as having:
   a. four total pregnancies, three full-term pregnancies, and one abortion
   b. four total pregnancies, three pregnancies to term, and one spontaneous abortion
   c. three total pregnancies, one full-term pregnancy, one abortion, and currently pregnant with twins
   d. four total pregnancies, three pregnancies to term, and one induced abortion

5. Every sonographer should be familiar with ultrasound-related organizations and suggested scanning protocols for their profession. Choose the group that will not provide reliable pelvic sonographic scanning information.
   a. AIUM
   b. ACR
   c. SDMS
   d. APR

6. An adequately filled bladder usually extends _____ the fundus of a nongravid uterus.
   a. slightly below
   b. at the same level of
   c. slightly beyond
   d. approximately 4 cm superior to

7. Select the correct optimization technique.
   a. Angle the sonographic beam parallel to the structure of interest.
   b. Use a lower-frequency transducer for penetration.
   c. Set focal zones 1 cm inferior to the structure of interest.
   d. Choose a low-frequency transducer for superficial structures.

8. If a premenopausal female should prepare for a gynecologic ultrasound by drinking 32 ounces of water 1 hour before the examination, what preparation would be suggested for a 70-year-old with vaginal bleeding and incontinence?
   a. No water preparation is needed.
   b. Approximately 10 ounces
   c. Approximately 25 ounces
   d. Approximately 50 ounces

9. A 2.5-MHz transducer is usually required to produce a diagnostic image on _____ patient.
   a. a large habitus
   b. an elderly
   c. a thin
   d. a 7-year-old

10. Endovaginal optimal focal range is from:
    a. 1 to 5 cm
    b. 2 to 7 cm
    c. the internal os to the uterine fundus
    d. the fornices to the uterine fundus

11. An optimal endovaginal image with the finest resolution possible can be created by:
    a. decreasing sector size
    b. using a 2.5-MHz transducer
    c. deepest depth setting
    d. requiring the patient to obtain a distended urinary bladder

12. Endovaginal transducers cannot be inserted past the area of the:
    a. vaginal fornices
    b. proximal urinary bladder
    c. distal vagina
    d. labia minora

13. Endovaginal ultrasound may not produce a diagnostic image in a patient:
    a. suspected of suffering with ovarian torsion
    b. who is being monitored for follicle size/ovulation
    c. with an enlarged leiomyomatous uterus
    d. scheduled for ova aspiration

14. Select the incorrect statement. Transperineal scanning:
    a. is a safe option to replace endovaginal imaging in the case of pregnancy with ruptured membranes
    b. images inferior to bowel gas, therefore avoiding obstructive shadows
    c. may be performed if a patient declines endovaginal scanning
    d. is performed between the labia on the perineum

15. Prior to an endovaginal ultrasound, the transducer should be lubricated. Which lubricant is best for a patient being treated for infertility?
    a. K-Y jelly
    b. None
    c. Saline
    d. Coupling gel

16. The sonographer can adjust power levels and scan efficiently to minimize patient exposure levels. This is known as:
    a. AIUM
    b. ARALA
    c. ALARA
    d. NIH guidelines

17. An ultrasound measurement of tissue stiffness is known as:
    a. displacement sonography
    b. compression sonography
    c. sonoelastography
    d. qualitative sonography

18. Individuals choosing sonography as a profession should become certified. The gold standard certifying body is:
    a. ARDMS
    b. ARRT
    c. AIUM
    d. RDMS

19. Sonohysterography images may demonstrate all except:
    a. patent fallopian tubes
    b. microbubbles within the uterine cavity
    c. endometrial polyps
    d. pelvic endometriosis

20. Mechanical acquisition volume transducers providing sequential still images use _____ planes.
    a. two
    b. three
    c. four
    d. three planes and the dimension of time

Fill-in-the-Blank

1. Prior to starting a patient sonographic examination, the sonographer should use _____ facility-accepted identifiers to confirm the patient's identification.

2. Optimization of an examination reduces costs and adheres to the _____ principle in reducing exposure to ultrasound energy and decreases patient discomfort.

3. A connected hospital can offer electronic systems such as HIS (_____), RIS (_____), EMR (_____), and MWL (_____) which will make a sonographer's job easier through the elimination of errors.

4. A full urinary bladder is necessary for a(n) _____ diagnostic pelvic examination, and an empty urinary bladder is necessary for a(n) _____ diagnostic pelvic exam.

5. A _____ requires a sonographer to place their hand on a patient's pelvic area while applying pressure in the region of the area of interest.

6. _____ refers to the number of previous pregnancies and includes the current gestation.

7. Parity of 3 (P3) refers to the number of pregnancies a woman has carried to _____.

8. _____ the transvaginal/endovaginal transducer prior to insertion to decrease patient discomfort.

9. The best resolution occurs within the _____ zone of the transducer.

10. Base your transducer choice on patient _____ and examination objectives.

11. _____ array transducers combine the wider field of view of sector transducers with greater near-field visualization and increased linear measurement accuracy.

12. If endovaginal scanning is contraindicated, the _____ approach may enable the sonographer to obtain images of the _____ and lower uterine segment.

13. Transvaginal/endovaginal ultrasound can assist in determining early detection of _____ pregnancy, diagnosis of placenta _____, and determination of fetal ____ rate and viability.

14. Imaging with 2D, color, and spectral Doppler is called _____ imaging.

15. Positioning the patient in a left or right _____ position may be helpful in the case of a less than optimally filled bladder when examining the female pelvis.

16. A ____-degree counterclockwise rotation of the transducer allows for imaging in transverse or oblique transverse planes.

17. A hysterosalpingogram (HSG) uses _____ as a contrast agent.

18. When imaging a solid ovarian mass, careful examination of the liver edge, flanks for _____, cul-de-sac, and _____ pouch is necessary.

19. _____-filled structures enhance the transmission of sound.

20. Ovarian size may be determined by measuring the ovary in ____ dimensions on views obtained in ____ orthogonal planes with calculation of the ovarian volume as necessary.

Short Answer

1. State pertinent clinical information that should be included in an ultrasound report.

2. Explain how a mass should be imaged, measured, and characterized.

3. Why is a filled bladder necessary for a transabdominal pelvic ultrasound and an empty bladder crucial to an endovaginal pelvic ultrasound?

IMAGE EVALUATION/PATHOLOGY

Answer the following questions.

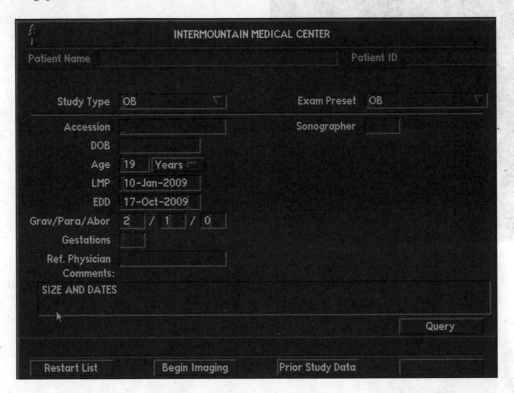

1. State the patient's identifiers on the PDE. How many pregnancies has this patient had? And how many children?

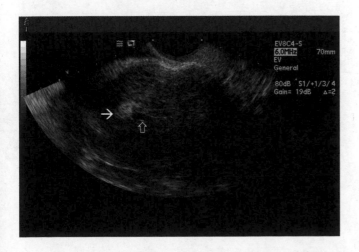

2. Describe what is visualized at the arrow and the open arrow.

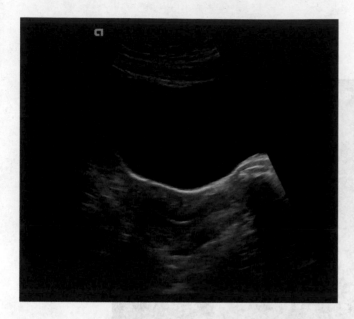

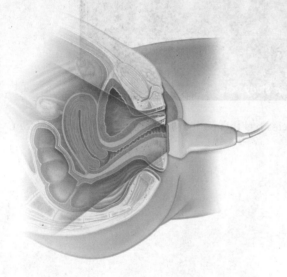

3. Explain what portion of the body is seen in the top, bottom, right, and left on the sagittal image.

4. What is the type of imaging method in this diagram?

CHAPTER 4

Obstetric Scanning Primer

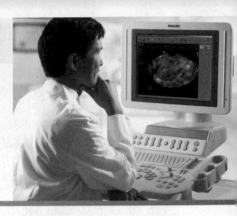

REVIEW OF GLOSSARY TERMS

Matching

Match the key terms with their definitions.

KEY TERMS

1. _____ placenta previa

2. _____ ectopic pregnancy

3. _____ thermal indices (TIs)

4. _____ vasa previa

5. _____ mechanical indices (MIs)

6. _____ aortocaval compression syndrome (supine hypotensive syndrome)

DEFINITION

a. Compression of the aorta and inferior vena cava (IVC) by the gravid uterus resulting in symptoms of nausea, hypotension, lightheadedness, and syncope

b. Entrapment of the umbilical cord between the presenting fetal part and the cervix

c. Pregnancy outside of the uterus

d. The amount of transmitted energy by the ultrasound beam. The higher the frequency, the lower the mechanical index (MI), thus, the lower the frequency, the higher the MI

e. Condition where the placenta implantation is low in the uterus and will deliver before the fetus

f. The output power indication of the amount of acoustic power it takes to raise the temperature of tissue by 1 °C

CHAPTER REVIEW

Multiple Choice

Complete each question by circling the best answer.

1. A moderately distended bladder is appropriate for obstetric imaging in:
   a. the second trimester and third trimester
   b. the first trimester
   c. all three trimesters
   d. the first and second trimesters

2. The inability of some females to lay supine during weeks 20-term of pregnancy because of a hypotensive state is known as:
   a. syncopal syndrome
   b. multiple gestation syndrome
   c. hypotensive compression syndrome
   d. aortocaval compression syndrome

3. A _____transducer may provide optimal images well into the third trimester on a thin patient.
   a. 2.5-MHz
   b. 3.5-MHz
   c. 5.0-MHz
   d. 7.5-MHz

4. Endovaginal transducers aid the clinician in determining all except:
   a. the presence of adnexal fluid resulting from an ectopic pregnancy
   b. fluid in Morison pouch
   c. gestational age in early pregnancy
   d. viability in early pregnancy

5. Choose the association that does not research and report on the safety of exposure to diagnostic ultrasound during pregnancy:
   a. FDA
   b. AIUM
   c. NIH
   d. ACR

6. A sonographer can adjust power levels and minimize patient exposure to diagnostic ultrasound by knowing and watching the ultrasound system ___ levels.
   a. NEMA
   b. both c and d
   c. TI
   d. MI

7. Select the correct statement.
   a. Adjusting MI, TI, output power, and persistence will maintain patient safety within ALARA guidelines.
   b. A 5.0-MHz transducer provides better depth penetration than a 3.5-MHz transducer.
   c. If the fetal kidneys and spine are positioned anteriorly in the gestational sac, select a lower-frequency transducer for the best imaging resolution.
   d. The output from Doppler (spectral and color) instruments tends to be lower than for gray-scale imaging.

8. Vasa previa means:
   a. a vessel leading to the uterus
   b. a reaction caused by compression of the uterus onto the aorta
   c. placenta covering the internal cervical os
   d. umbilical cord is positioned between the internal cervical os and a fetal part

9. An SPTA below _____ mW/cm^2 for an unfocused beam decreases the possibility of bioeffects.
   a. 10
   b. 50
   c. 100
   d. 500

10. A correctly filled bladder allows for imaging of the _____ and the lower placental edge.
    a. placenta
    b. cervix
    c. presenting part
    d. cesarean section scar

Fill-in-the-Blank

1. Aortocaval syndrome results in maternal feelings of nausea and dizziness owing to compression of the _____ and _____.

2. Doppler ultrasound in the _____ trimester should be used only when medically indicated.

3. High _____ and _____ increase potential bioeffects to the embryo and fetus.

4. A _____ evaluation of the uterus helps in imaging for retained products of conception or abnormal clotting.

5. To limit effects of aortocaval compression syndrome, position a support under the patient's _____ so that scanning can be completed.

6. Imaging a pregnant patient before the 15th week of gestation requires the same technique as a _____ ultrasound examination.

7. In the first trimester, transabdominal imaging requires a full bladder to push the air-filled _____ out of the false pelvis and allow for an unobstructed view of the uterus.

8. ALARA means _____.

Short Answer

1. Discuss an organized routine for scanning a second- and third-trimester ultrasound examination anatomical study.

2. What is "prudent use" regarding obstetric sonography as defined by the AIUM?

3. Suggest patient management techniques for relieving hypotension during an obstetric ultrasound examination.

IMAGE EVALUATION/PATHOLOGY

Answer the following questions.

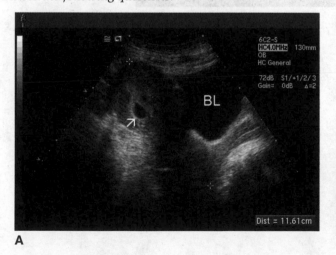

A

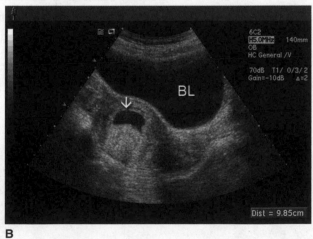

B

1. Does image A or image B show a fully distended bladder?

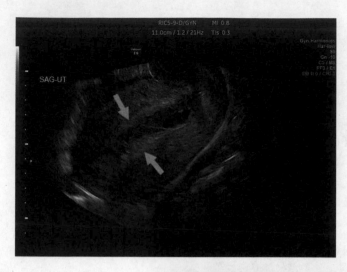

2. a. Does the image display a normal postpartum endometrium?

   b. Discuss the appropriate transducer for and post-partum uterus with clotting and bloody discharge.

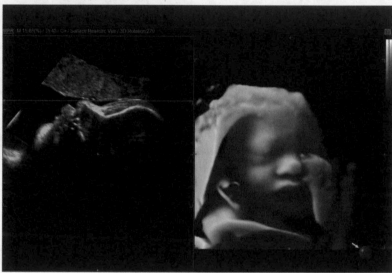

3. Name the type of ultrasound used in the left image. Name the type of image and the technique used in the right image.

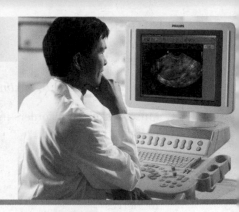

CHAPTER 5

Foundational Ultrasound Ergonomics for Obstetrics and Gynecology

REVIEW OF GLOSSARY TERMS

Matching

Match the key terms with their definitions.

KEY TERMS

1. _____ extension

2. _____ lordosis

3. _____ repetition

4. _____ static posture

5. _____ risk factor

6. _____ hyperextension

7. _____ abduction

8. _____ flexion

9. _____ neutral position

10. _____ ergonomics

11. _____ posture

12. _____ workstation

13. _____ repetitive stress injury

DEFINITION

a. Any behavior that increases the chances of developing MSKD

b. The creation of a safe workplace that involves the sonographer and ultrasound system positioning

c. Movement beyond the normal range of a joint

d. A position that increases the angle of a joint (i.e., the unbending of the elbow, straightening of the spine)

e. The position of our bodies

f. Fixed or unchanging position

g. Excessive anterior curvature of the spine

h. Work area encompassing the equipment (i.e., ultrasound system, patient bed)

i. Repeated movements. When coupled with force and awkward body positions increase the risk of MSKD development

j. The decrease of an angle of a joint (i.e., bending of the elbow, curling of the spine)

k. Cumulative injury caused by repeated movement of a musculoskeletal structure

l. Moving away from the center of the body

m. Body position without flexion or extension

CHAPTER REVIEW

Multiple Choice

Complete each question by circling the best answer.

1. Musculoskeletal disorders involve all except injury to the:
   a. ligaments
   b. acromion
   c. tendons
   d. nerves

2. The most common location for WRMSK pain in a sonographer involves the:
   a. back
   b. wrist
   c. neck
   d. shoulder

3. A chronic work injury displays these signs:
   a. aching, fatigue, stiffness, muscle or joint discomfort, and pain
   b. aching, fatigue, stiffness, and muscle or joint discomfort
   c. aching, fatigue, stiffness, muscle or joint discomfort, pain, plus weakness or inability to hold objects
   d. aching, fatigue, stiffness, muscle or joint discomfort, and headache

4. One of the largest risk factors for MSKD is:
   a. circulation reduction
   b. an awkward body position
   c. maintaining a neutral spine
   d. decreased reach

5. The ultrasound system monitor should be positioned approximately ___ inches from the sonographer's face and eyes.
   a. 20
   b. 30
   c. 40
   d. 50

6. Transducer cable twisting and weight can cause torque on a sonographer's wrist. Select the best way to remedy wrist torque.
   a. Use cable supports.
   b. Adjust control panel height.
   c. Adjust chair height.
   d. Rotate the monitor.

7. Choose the correct ergonomic statement.
   a. Limit portable examinations that require static or awkward positions and forceful transducer handling.
   b. Maintain scanning position.
   c. Schedule like exam types together (i.e., abdominal in the morning, obstetrics in the afternoon).
   d. Use similar motions for each examination.

8. Choose the correct wrist position for maintaining a healthy ergonomic position.
   a. Radial deviated
   b. Neutral
   c. Ventrally flexed
   d. Dorsally extended

9. Select a cause for an unhealthy forceful transducer grip:
   a. patient breathing
   b. decreased carpal muscle integrity
   c. lighter equipment
   d. patient obesity

10. Choose the correct suggested rest break to relieve muscle tension and increase joint and muscle flow during an extended ultrasound examination:
    a. 1-minute break every 10 minutes
    b. 30- to 60-second mini-break every 20 minutes
    c. 1-minute break every hour
    d. 30-second mini-break every 5 minutes

Fill-in-the-Blank

1. MSKDs are the result of accumulated _____ over a prolonged time.

2. WRMSKD means _____.

3. Patient _____ has led to the use of increasing axial force to acquire diagnostic images.

4. Most ultrasound systems allow for independent monitor positioning, _____, _____, and _____, providing a method to decrease neck flexion and extension.

5. It is known that WRMSKDs are a _____ process involving both personal and work behaviors.

6. With the overuse of the wrist, swelling occurs, compressing nerves and tendons, increasing the risk of developing _____ and _____.

7. The most ergonomic sitting position is when the forearms and thighs are _____ to the floor.

8. When sitting to perform an ultrasound examination, the feet should be _____.

9. To decrease the chance of developing back pain while scanning, maintain _____ spine alignment.

10. Features of an ergonomic chair that will aid with controlling work injuries are _____, _____, and _____.

Short Answer

1. List the work tasks that increase the potential for muscular injury.

2. Discuss demands in the work environment that a sonographer may not control and increases the risk of injury.

3. Maintaining neutral reach zones links to a balanced spine and decreased WRMSKS. Explain the horizontal and vertical neutral zones.

4. Offer suggestions to minimize force when force is used to move the ultrasound system for a portable examination.

IMAGE EVALUATION/PATHOLOGY

Answer the following questions.

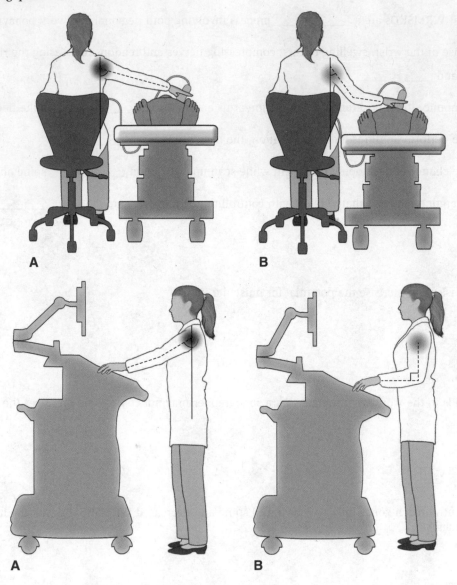

A   B

A   B

1. Choose the arm position that will cause less fatigue and pain.

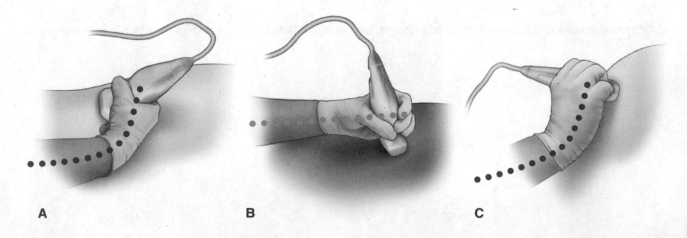

A   B   C

2. What is the best wrist position to alleviate pain and muscle fatigue?

PART TWO

GYNECOLOGIC SONOGRAPHY

CHAPTER 6

Embryonic Development of the Female Genital System

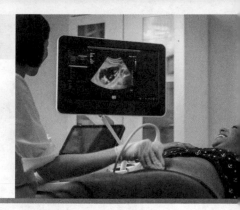

REVIEW OF GLOSSARY TERMS

Matching

Match the key terms with their definitions.

KEY TERMS

1. _____ mesonephros (wolffian ducts)

2. _____ hydronephrosis

3. _____ oogonia

4. _____ urogenital

5. _____ gonadal ridges

6. _____ müllerian ducts (paramesonephric ducts)

7. _____ broad ligament

8. _____ pronephros

9. _____ allantois

10. _____ embryogenesis

11. _____ hydroureter

12. _____ mesonephric ducts

13. _____ primordial germ cells

14. _____ atretic

15. _____ oocytes

16. _____ diploid

17. _____ hydrometrocolpos

18. _____ mesovarium

19. _____ cloaca

DEFINITION

a. Large, sometimes tortuous ureter because of distal blockage

b. Second stage of kidney development (aka wolffian body)

c. Connection between the mesonephros and the cloaca

d. Structure that appears at approximately 5 weeks gestation that becomes either ovaries or testes

e. Blockage or absence of a structure

f. Immature oocytes

g. Pertaining to the urinary and genital system

h. Sac-like vascular structure that lies below the chorion and develops from the hindgut

i. Accumulation of secreted fluid resulting in distention of the uterus and vagina because of obstruction

j. Fold of peritoneum that connects the uterus to the pelvis

k. Cavity that is part of the development of the digestive and reproductive organs

l. Paired ducts that become the oviducts, uterus, cervix, and upper vagina

m. Section of the uterine broad ligament that covers the ovary

n. Formation of an embryo

o. Primary or first kidney that develops in the embryo

p. Precursor of germ cells, become oocytes or spermatozoa in the adult

q. Urine collection in the kidneys because of distal obstruction

r. Female germ cells

s. Normal number of paired chromosomes

ANATOMY AND PHYSIOLOGY REVIEW

Image Labeling

Complete the labels in the images that follow.

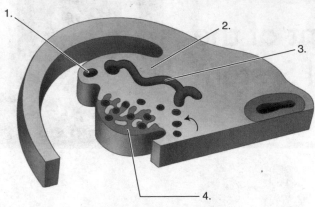

Primitive sex cords

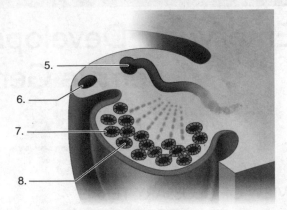

Primitive germ cells differentiate into oogonia

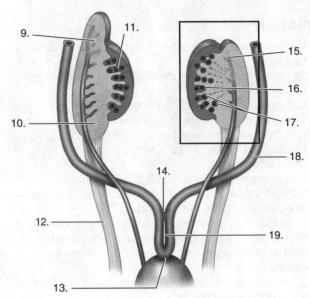

Female müllerian ductal system

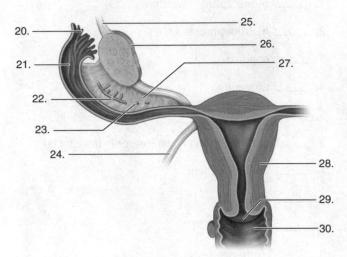

Female pelvic organs

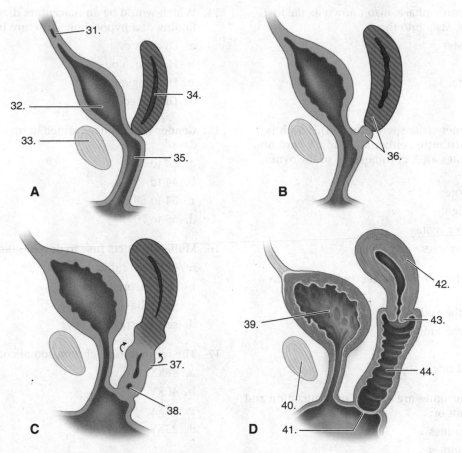

Female organ formation

CHAPTER REVIEW

Multiple Choice

Complete each question by circling the best answer.

1. A method used to classify the embryo, placing the embryo into categories depending on age, size, and morphologic characteristics, is called:
   a. organism staging
   b. Carnegie staging
   c. fetal staging
   d. neonatal staging

2. Fetal period genitourinary anomalies include all except:
   a. ureter agenesis
   b. hydrometrocolpos
   c. pre-embryonic fusion
   d. obstructive uropathy

3. Cloacal anomalies can result in:
   a. bicornuate uterus
   b. renal cysts
   c. intra-abdominal lesions
   d. hydrometrocolpos

4. An ultrasound examination of a patient with hematocolpos should include imaging of the:
   a. kidneys
   b. liver
   c. spleen
   d. pancreas

5. The most common mass lesions in neonates are of:
   a. renal origin
   b. intestinal origin
   c. pulmonary origin
   d. peritoneal origin

6. Often development abnormalities in the female pelvis become apparent:
   a. when primigravida
   b. during the standard Level 2 Obstetric ultrasound
   c. at the onset of puberty
   d. at the onset of a UTI (urinary tract infection)

7. The pre-embryonic phase, also known as the first Carnegie stage, lasts into the:
   a. third trimester
   b. first week
   c. first trimester
   d. third week

8. If the male gamete (the spermatozoon), which is capable of contributing either an X or a Y chromosome, contributes an X chromosome to the ovum, the result is:
   a. a male zygote
   b. a female zygote
   c. twin female zygotes
   d. twin male zygotes

9. Precursors to the female ovaries and to the male testes:
   a. arise from the yolk sac
   b. arise from the kidneys
   c. are diploid
   d. are gonadal ridges

10. Diploid chromosomes are a result of fertilization and result in a count of:
    a. 23 chromosomes
    b. 13 chromosomes
    c. 46 chromosomes
    d. 18 chromosomes

11. What cells produce a gender appearance?
    a. Primordial germ cells
    b. Ectoderm cells
    c. Gonadal germ cells
    d. Mesoderm cells

12. At birth, there are approximately _____ oogonia in the female newborn.
    a. 7 million
    b. 1 million
    c. 500,000
    d. 300 to 400

13. The vaginal fornices surround the end of the:
    a. distal vaginal canal
    b. labia
    c. hymen
    d. cervix

14. Which would be an inaccurate diagnosis for the finding of a hypoechoic structure in the fetal pelvis?
    a. Ovarian cyst
    b. Hematocolpos
    c. Hemangioma
    d. Distended bladder

15. Gender (sex) is determined at *approximately* _____ days.
    a. 28 to 32
    b. 44 to 49
    c. 54 to 58
    d. 66 to 70

16. Müllerian ducts fuse to develop the uterus and:
    a. fallopian tubes
    b. suspensory ligament
    c. genitalia
    d. second-stage kidneys

17. The normal male chromosomal configuration is:
    a. 46XX
    b. 46XY
    c. 23XX
    d. 23XY

18. What hormone is absent in the female fetus that causes regression of the mesonephric ducts?
    a. Maternal estrogen
    b. Male inducer substance
    c. Placental estrogen
    d. Circulating teste hormone

19. What systems develop in tandem in the embryo and are still closely associated in the adult?
    a. Pulmonary and circulatory
    b. Urinary and musculoskeletal
    c. Reproductive and urinary
    d. Respiratory and digestive

20. Hydronephrosis and hydroureter can display as a mass in the fetal:
    a. cervix
    b. chest
    c. ovary
    d. pelvis

Fill-in-the-Blank

1. In the first few months of early development, the _____ are undifferentiated.

2. External development of genitalia is similar in both sexes until approximately the _____ week.

3. The promoting factor in the development of female external genitalia is maternal _____.

4. Bartholin and Skene glands, the clitoris, _____ minora and _____, vestibule, vagina, and mons _____ make up the external genitalia.

5. The _____ becomes the genital tubercle in both genders.

6. Gonadal gender can be determined in the _____ embryo at approximately the _____ day of gestation, which correlates with Carnegie stage 18.

7. Carnegie stage 20 correlates to day 49 for gonadal gender in the _____ embryo.

8. The first-stage kidney known as _____ forms during the fifth week, and second-stage kidney known as _____ form in the sixth week.

9. Müllerian ducts fuse to develop the normal _____, also giving rise to the _____.

10. The _____ and _____ systems develop simultaneously, resulting in coexisting malformations.

11. Determination of chromosomal gender or sex occurs at the time of _____.

12. Vaginal formation occurs through development of the _____ sinus and the primitive _____.

13. The ovary is suspended by the _____, the _____ ligament of the ovary, and the _____ ligament.

14. Most congenital anomalies in fetuses in utero occur in the genitourinary system, with urinary tract abnormalities accounting for about _____ of the total.

15. The female gamete, known as the ovum, contributes to the _____ chromosome.

16. Embryogenesis is formation of an _____.

17. Between puberty and menopause, approximately _____ to _____ fertile ova are produced.

18. If an abnormal fluid collection is suspected in utero in the midline female pelvis, _____ outflow may be obstructed.

19. A female gonad is a(n) _____.

20. Prenatal ultrasound may also detect congenital anomalies in the ovaries, uterus, and vagina, especially when they enlarge and produce a pelvic _____.

Short Answer

1. Describe how hydrometrocolpos would appear on fetal ultrasound.

2. Name and briefly describe the four ligaments of the female pelvis.

3. Excited first-time parents (primigravida) are presenting for an ultrasound for unsure dates. The mother has a large body habitus and a history of irregular cycles, of which she does not record dates. They are thrilled to view the pregnancy images and are hoping to learn the fetal gender. Endovaginal ultrasound was performed because of maternal body habitus, and calculations date the fetus at 9w2d (9 weeks 2 days). Can gender information be provided to the parents and why?

CHAPTER 7

Congenital Anomalies of the Female Genital System

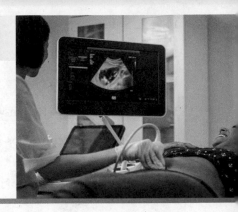

REVIEW OF GLOSSARY TERMS

Matching

Match the key terms with their definitions.

KEY TERMS

1. _____ metroplasty

2. _____ uterine aplasia

3. _____ ostium (pl. ostia)

4. _____ hematocolpos

5. _____ imperforate hymen

6. _____ apoptosis

7. _____ renal agenesis

8. _____ hydrometra

9. _____ Klippel-Feil syndrome

10. _____ uterus unicornis unicollis

11. _____ diethylstilbestrol (DES)

12. _____ hymen

13. _____ cervical incompetence

DEFINITION

a. Anomaly that results in one vagina, two cervices, and two uterine horns

b. Mechanism by which the uterine septum regresses

c. Accumulation of watery fluid in the uterine cavity

d. Uterus didelphys with obstructed unilateral vagina and associated ipsilateral renal and ureter agenesis

e. Retention of blood in the uterine cavity

f. Paired embryonic tubes roughly parallel with the mesonephric ducts that empty into the urogenital sinus; in the female, the upper part of these ducts forms the fallopian tubes and the lower parts fuse to form the uterus

g. Congenital anomalies of the vertebra/anus/cardiac/trachea/esophagus/radius/renal/limb of unknown etiology

h. A small opening, especially one of entrance into a hollow organ or canal, such as the fallopian tube

i. Complete failure of resorption of the uterovaginal septum

j. Medical condition in which a pregnant woman's cervix begins to dilate and efface before her pregnancy has reached term. This may cause miscarriage or preterm birth during the second and third trimesters.

k. Characterized by congenital fusion of the cervical spine, a short neck, a low posterior hairline, and limited range of cervical spine motion. Associated with Mayer-Rokitansky-Küster-Hauser syndrome

l. Anomaly that results in one cervix and one uterine horn

m. Nonsteroidal drug administered between the late 1940s to early 1970s to pregnant women. This drug was first demonstrated as a transplacental carcinogen responsible for clear-cell vaginal carcinoma in girls born to mothers who took the drug during pregnancy to prevent miscarriage. Uterine malformations associated with this drug's exposure include uterine hypoplasia and a T-shaped endometrium.

14. _____ hematometra

15. _____ congenital

16. _____ uterine didelphys

17. _____ Wunderlich-Herlyn-Werner syndrome

18. _____ hematometrocolpos

19. _____ uterus arcuate

20. _____ sinovaginal bulb

21. _____ paramesonephric (müllerian) ducts

22. _____ uterus bicornis bicollis

23. _____ septate uterus

24. _____ hysterosalpingography

25. _____ uterine bicornis unicollis

26. _____ subseptate uterus

27. _____ VATER/VACTERL syndrome

n. Reconstructive surgery on the uterus for women with reproductive failure
o. Accumulation of menstrual blood in the uterus and vagina caused by either an imperforate hymen or other obstruction
p. Mildest fusion anomaly, resulting in a partial indentation of the uterine fundus with a normal endometrial cavity; considered a normal variant
q. Anomaly that results in two vaginas, two cervices, and two uteri
r. Absence of one or both kidneys
s. Complete absence of the uterus
t. Radiographic imaging of the uterus and fallopian tubes after injection of radiopaque material
u. Partial failure of the medial septum to be reabsorbed
v. Anomaly that results in one vagina, one cervix, and two uterine horns
w. Part of the vaginal plate of the urogenital sinus, which forms the lower 20% of the vagina
x. Usually congenital owing to failure of degeneration of central epithelial cells of the hymenal membrane. An imperforate hymen is visible upon examination as a translucent thin membrane just inferior to the urethral meatus that bulges with the Valsalva maneuver and completely covers the vagina; it must be surgically corrected.
y. Ring-like area of tissue that represents the opening to the vagina
z. Accumulation of menstrual blood in the vagina resulting from a lower vaginal obstruction or imperforate hymen
aa. Mental or physical traits, anomalies, malformations, or diseases present at birth

ANATOMY AND PHYSIOLOGY REVIEW

Image Labeling

Complete the labels in the images that follow.

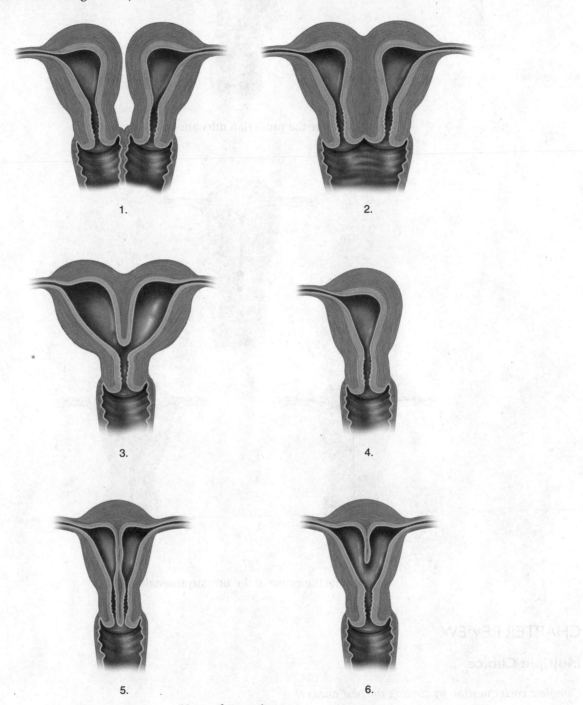

1.

2.

3.

4.

5.

6.

Name the uterine types.

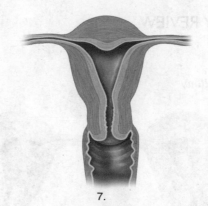

7.

Name the mullerian duct anomaly

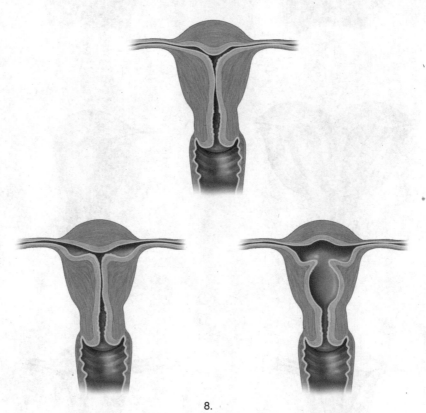

8.

Name the cause of the uterine anomaly.

CHAPTER REVIEW

Multiple Choice

Complete each question by circling the best answer.

1. Complications from uterine and vaginal malformations do not occur from:
   a. failure of resorption of median septum
   b. paramesonephric (müllerian) duct arrested development
   c. failure of fusion of the müllerian ducts
   d. distal ductal regression

2. Germ cells that migrate from the yolk sac to the gonadal region form the:
   a. genital ridges becoming sex cords
   b. mesonephric ducts
   c. female embryos
   d. fallopian tubes

3. Apoptosis is related to:
   a. DES
   b. regression of the uterine septum
   c. a short cervical neck
   d. paired embryonic tubes

4. Sonography is useful in imaging _____, a combination of menstrual blood, fluid, and secretions in the distended vagina and uterus caused by imperforate hymen.
   a. sinovaginal bulb
   b. amenorrhea
   c. hematometrocolpos
   d. neovagina

5. Arrested development of the bilateral müllerian ducts causes:
   a. hypoplasia of the uterus
   b. hypoplasia of the vagina
   c. hypoplasia of both the uterus and vagina
   d. uterus unicornis unicollis

6. MRKH and MURCS are related to:
   a. fetal renal and spinal anomalies
   b. a long fetal neck
   c. fetal hematometra
   d. a high hairline

7. The wolffian duct forms the sinovaginal bulbs which with the müllerian tubercle finally becomes:
   a. hymen
   b. lower one-fifth of the vagina
   c. complete vagina
   d. urogenital sinus

8. Uterine agenesis is imaged best in the:
   a. coronal plane
   b. parasagittal plane
   c. transverse plane
   d. sagittal plane

9. Defects of vertical vaginal fusion can result in the formation of a transverse vaginal septum, which can cause:
   a. uterine aplasia
   b. obstruction and hematocolpos
   c. functional vaginal endometrial tissue
   d. uterus arcuatus

10. Initially, a transverse vaginal septum requires all except:
    a. laparoscopy for endometriosis
    b. drainage of accumulated menstrual blood
    c. preservation of a perineal space of adequate size to function as a normal vagina
    d. septum excision

11. The easiest vaginal anomaly to view sonographically is:
    a. duplicated vagina
    b. transverse septum
    c. complete absence of the vagina
    d. longitudinal septa

12. Which imaging modality is extremely helpful if hematometrocolpos or hematometra distorts the reproductive organs causing limited imaging capability using ultrasound?
    a. Laparoscopy
    b. Transperineal sonography
    c. CT
    d. MRI

13. Sonohysterography is also known as:
    a. saline sonography (SS)
    b. 3D hysterography
    c. static hysterography
    d. saline-infused sonography (SIS)

14. Choose the most effective diagnostic method for determining uterus unicornis.
    a. 2D vaginal sonography
    b. HSG
    c. NM
    d. 2D abdominal sonography

15. Bicornuate uterus is related to:
    a. difficulty conceiving
    b. postdate delivery
    c. cervical incompetence
    d. vaginal incompetence

16. Choose a definite method for distinguishing bicornuate uterus from septate anomalies.
    a. MRI, 3D endovaginal sonography
    b. MRI, HSG
    c. HSG, 3D sonography
    d. HSG, 3D transabdominal sonography

17. Complete midline failure of müllerian duct fusion results in:
    a. septate uterus
    b. uterine didelphys
    c. bicornuate uterus
    d. unicornuate uterus

18. The uterine septum consists of:
    a. poorly vascularized fibromuscular tissue
    b. highly vascularized fibromuscular tissue
    c. nonvascular fibromuscular tissue
    d. muscular and connective tissue

19. Uterus didelphys, more than any other müllerian anomaly, is associated with:
    a. ovarian agenesis
    b. renal agenesis
    c. cervix agenesis
    d. vaginal agenesis

20. Anomalies of the fallopian tubes include:
    a. tube duplication, accessory ostia, and hypoplasia
    b. ectopic location and hyperplasia
    c. luminal atresia, absent muscular layer, and absent ampulla
    d. accessory ostia, patency, and double tube

Fill-in-the-Blank

1. Most congenital anomalies are diagnosed in the _____ or recurrent _____ loss populations.

2. It is extremely important to distinguish between a _____ and a septate uterus because the pregnancy outcomes and treatment techniques differ considerably.

3. DES-exposed women have uterine anomalies visualized with _____.

4. 3D multiplanar _____ sonography is valuable in imaging the hypoplastic uterus and T-shaped uterine cavity.

5. Fallopian tube patency can be established with _____ or _____ using a contrast agent or saline.

6. A double cervix (cervical duplication), in rare cases, develops with a complete _____ and _____ septa.

7. Pelvic ultrasound can help to diagnose _____, menstrual blood, fluid, and secretions in the uterus and vagina.

8. A _____ septum is not the same as the imperforate hymen.

9. The method used to create a vagina if vaginal agenesis is diagnosed is _____.

10. A mild indentation of the superior portion of the endometrium is called an _____ uterus.

11. In the case of atretic or absent vagina, the _____ scanning approach is helpful.

12. Uterus _____ is the result of normal development of half of the uterus with no or rudimentary development of the rest.

13. Sonographic _____ imaging of the unicornis uterus is sensitive, demonstrating myometrial and _____ structures, as well as cervical canal, uterine external contours, and cornual angles.

14. A bicornuate uterus _____ failed to fuse while a uterine didelphys _____ failed to fuse.

15. A _____ duct cyst is a very common remnant of the distal mesonephric duct.

16. Hematometra is retention of blood in the _____.

17. Narrowing of the uterine cavity by the septum is a condition suggesting poor _____ outcome.

18. HSG, _____, CT, and _____ help diagnose and monitor patients with congenital anomalies of the genital tract.

19. DES (diethylstilbestrol) is known to cause a _____ shaped uterine endometrium.

20. Ectopic ovaries are known as _____ or accessory.

Short Answer

1. A 16-year-old female complains of monthly pelvic pain. The physician learns that the patient has not begun menstruating. Upon physical examination, the physician notes a fullness in her inferior mid pelvis. What is the most likely diagnosis? Describe what ultrasound would demonstrate.

2. A 23-year-old with a bicornuate uterus miscarried her first pregnancy in the 18th week. She is currently 13 weeks pregnant. Discuss what can be done to increase the ability to continue this pregnancy to term. Explain why intervention may be necessary.

3. A 32-year-old DES-exposed woman was undergoing a hysterosalpingogram (HSG) because she had spontaneously aborted two times and had one ectopic pregnancy that resulted in the surgical loss of her right fallopian tube. Describe possible uterine findings the HSG will demonstrate.

IMAGE EVALUATION/PATHOLOGY

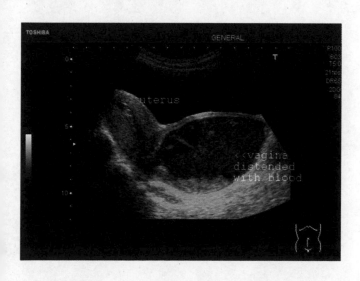

1. Name the imaged structure and view. What is the likely diagnosis?

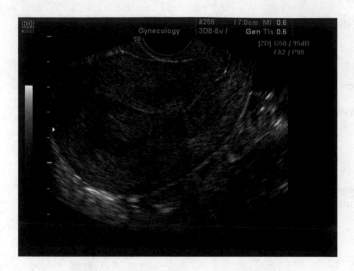

2. Name the imaged structure and view. Offer a diagnosis.

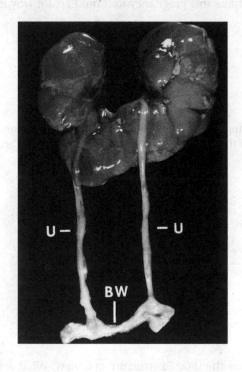

3. Explain the image. What organ is shown? U-ureter, BW-bladder wall.

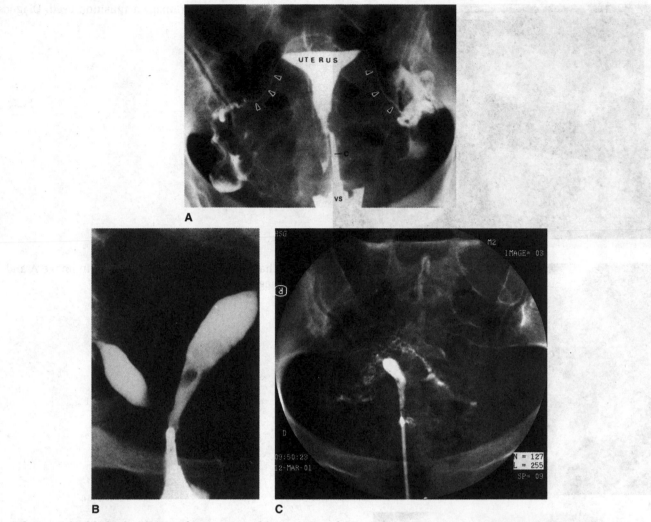

A

B   **C**

4. What are the likely diagnoses of image A and images B and C?

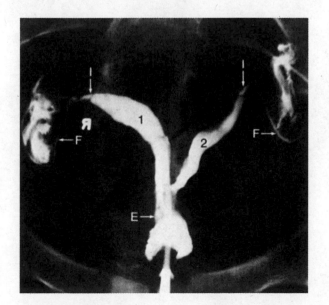

5. Name the uterine type.

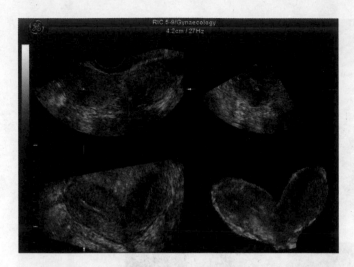

6. Explain the type of image acquisition used. Diagnose the uterine type.

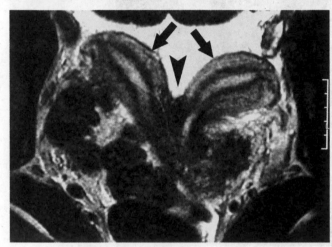

7. What is the type of uterine variant in image A and image B?

A

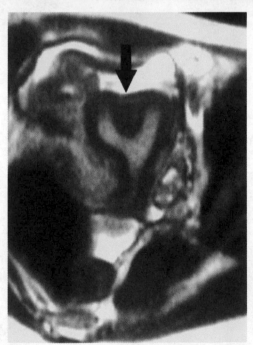

B

CHAPTER 8

The Female Cycle

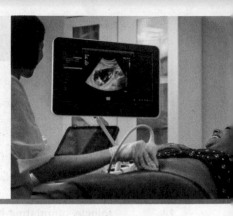

REVIEW OF GLOSSARY TERMS

Matching

Match the key terms with their definitions.

KEY TERMS

1. _____ antrum (follicular)

2. _____ theca interna

3. _____ positive feedback loop

4. _____ luteinization

5. _____ corpus luteum (Latin for "yellow body")

6. _____ progesterone

7. _____ amenorrhea

8. _____ gonadotropic protein

9. _____ retroverted

10. _____ estrogen

11. _____ menorrhagia

12. _____ negative feedback

13. _____ dysmenorrhea

14. _____ oligomenorrhea

15. _____ suspensory (infundibulopelvic) ligament

16. _____ theca externa

17. _____ cardinal ligament

DEFINITION

a. Absence of menstruation

b. Male hormones produced in small quantities by the female ovaries and adrenal glands, with the greatest quantities occurring at the midpoint of a woman's menstrual cycle

c. An outer layer of a mature follicle containing spindle-shaped cells that are incapable of hormone production

d. Uterus angled forward toward the cervix

e. Forward-tipped uterus with the cervix and vaginal canal forming a 90-degree angle or less

f. The portion of an ovarian follicle filled with liquor folliculi. Spaces formed by the confluence of small lakes of follicular liquid in the ovary

g. Regulates the release of FSH and LH by gonadotropes from the anterior pituitary

h. Painful menstruation

i. A system of glands and cells that produce hormones released directly in the circulatory system

j. General term for female steroid sex hormones secreted by the ovary and responsible for female sexual characteristics

k. Hormone produced by the anterior pituitary, which stimulates ovarian follicle production in females and sperm production in males

l. Hormones secreted by the gonadotrope cells of the pituitary gland

m. Endocrine cells located in the anterior pituitary that produce the gonadotropins; examples are follicle-stimulating hormone (FSH) and luteinizing hormone.

n. A mature, fully developed ovarian cyst containing the ripe ovum

o. The transformation of the mature ovarian follicle into a corpus luteum

18. _____ endocrine system

19. _____ anteverted

20. _____ mesometrium

21. _____ gonadotrope cell

22. _____ rectouterine recess (pouch)

23. _____ anteflexed

24. _____ follicle-stimulating hormone (FSH)

25. _____ retroflexed

26. _____ Graafian follicle

27. _____ perimetrium

28. _____ broad ligament

29. _____ polymenorrhea (poly = many, menorrhea = bleeding)

30. _____ androgen

31. _____ gonadotropin-releasing hormone (GnRH)

p. When concentration of a hormone rises above a certain level, a series of actions take place within a system to cause the concentration to fall. Conversely, steps are taken to increase concentration when the level is too low.

q. Abnormally heavy or prolonged menstruation

r. The mesentery of the uterus. It constitutes the majority of the broad ligament of the uterus, excluding only the portions adjacent to the uterine tube and ovary

s. Abnormally light or infrequent menstruation. Opposite of menorrhagia

t. Outer serosal layer of the uterus, equivalent to peritoneum

u. Steps taken to increase concentration when a level is too low

v. Frequent irregular periods

w. A steroid hormone produced by the corpus luteum, whose function is to prepare and maintain the endometrium for the reception and development of the fertilized ovum

x. Area in the pelvic cavity between the rectum and the uterus that is likely to accumulate free fluid; also known as the posterior cul-de-sac and the pouch of Douglas

y. A backward angle of the uterine fundus in relation to the cervix

z. A uterus tilted posterior towards the rectum

aa. A peritoneum ligament extending upward from the upper pole of the ovary

bb. A vascular ovarian layer characterized by polyhedral cells that secrete estrogen. The cells are developed from stromal cells, which produce steroid hormones

cc. The ligament with a peritoneal fold that also supports the fallopian tubes, uterus, and vagina. It connects the sides of the uterus to the walls and floor of the pelvis.

dd. The ligament that attaches to the uterus at the level of the cervix and from the superior part of the vagina to the lateral walls of the pelvis. The cardinal ligament provides support to the uterus.

ee. Formed in the ovary when a follicle has matured and released its egg (ovum) after ovulation. The follicle becomes the corpus luteum that produces progesterone. Progesterone causes the lining of the uterus to thicken for egg implantation.

ANATOMY AND PHYSIOLOGY REVIEW

Image Labeling

Complete the labels in the images that follow.

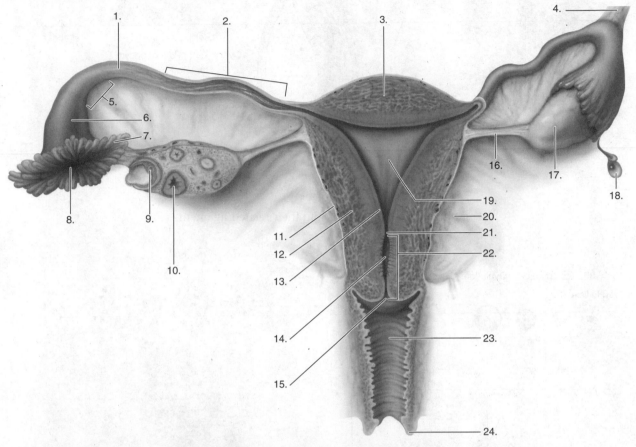

Anatomy of the female reproductive system

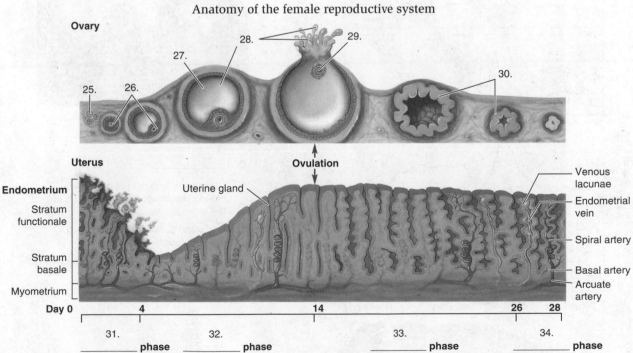

Ovarian and endometrial cycle association

Interconnectivity between ovarian and endometrial cycle association through the menstrual cycle.

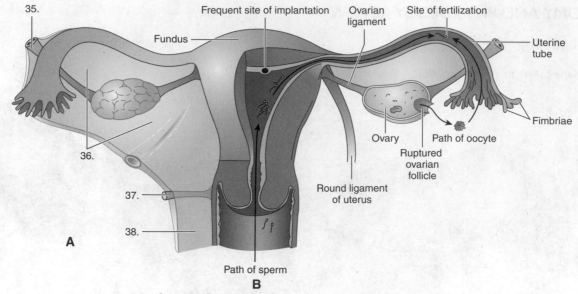

Female reproductive organs and their related ligaments

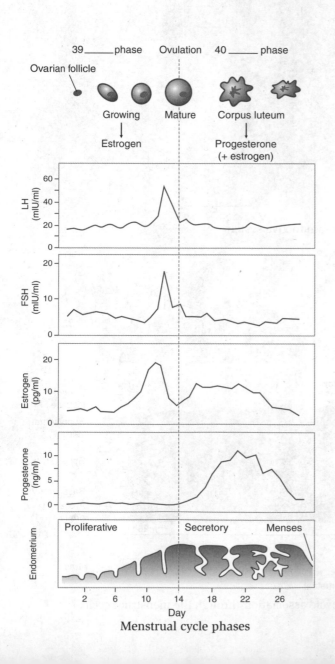

Menstrual cycle phases

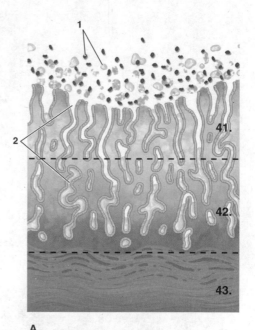

A _____

B _____

C _____

1 Uterine cavity with epithelial cells, blood corpuscles, and remainders of the expulsed mucosa

2 Intact and partially expulsed uterine glands

Endometrial layers during menstruation.

CHAPTER REVIEW

Multiple Choice

Complete each question by circling the best answer.

1. Which is not a uterine layer?
   a. Myometrium
   b. Endometrium
   c. Serometrium
   d. Perimetrium

2. Changes in the endometrium, which constitutes the menstrual cycle, are preparation for:
   a. fertilization of the oocyte
   b. fertilized ovum arrival
   c. luteinizing phase
   d. secretory phase

3. Female reproductive cycle is defined as:
   a. span from menarche (beginning of menstrual function) to menopause (cessation of menstrual function)
   b. span beginning with the fertilized ovum through birth
   c. the ovarian and uterine cycles, the hormonal changes that regulate them, and related cyclical changes in the breasts and cervix
   d. premenses and postmenopause

4. Endometrial sloughing is caused by:
   a. increasing levels of estrogen
   b. increasing levels of progesterone
   c. decreasing levels of estrogen
   d. decreasing levels of progesterone

5. Which statement correctly describes fallopian tube anatomy?
   a. The widest portion of the fallopian tube is the isthmus.
   b. The fimbriae connect to the uterine cornua.
   c. The infundibulum is the distal funnel-shaped portion of the fallopian tube.
   d. The isthmus contains finger-like projections called fimbriae.

6. Normal ovaries are oval shaped and measure approximately:
   a. 5 × 3 × 15 mm
   b. 5 × 5 × 3 mm
   c. 2 × 3 × 4 in
   d. 5 × 3 × 1.5 cm

7. The lowest portion of the uterus is the:
   a. vagina
   b. external os
   c. internal os
   d. cervix

8. Endocrine hormones secreted by the hypothalamus control reproductive events. Choose which is not related to the female cycle:
   a. GnRH
   b. LH
   c. FSH
   d. CCK

9. Designate the cranial structure that is essential for survival and reproduction:
   a. hypothalamus
   b. endocrine system
   c. diencephalon
   d. thalamus

10. Secondary amenorrhea is described as:
    a. women who have started menstruation then had an absence of their menses for three cycles or 6 months
    b. infrequent or light menstruation
    c. failure of menstruation to begin
    d. transient, intermittent, or permanent cessation of menstruation

11. Select the correct statement
    a. Ovaries increase estrogen production during menopause.
    b. Menopause and postmenopause are interchangeable terms.
    c. Polycystic ovarian syndrome (PCOS) causes frequent menstruation.
    d. PCOS is related to anovulation.

12. Amenorrhea is:
    a. irregular menstruation
    b. absence of menstruation
    c. heavy menstruation
    d. spotty menstruation

13. Hormone replacement therapy may cause:
    a. maintenance of ovarian volume
    b. decreased ovarian volume
    c. absent folliculogenesis
    d. menopause

14. The luteal phase:
    a. begins during ovulation
    b. begins after ovulation
    c. begins approximately day 28 of the cycle
    d. needs to be at least 5 days duration to allow for a healthy implantation

15. Choose the function that FSH is not involved with.
    a. Progression of the menstrual cycle
    b. Spermatogenesis in men
    c. Ovarian follicle development
    d. Ova maturation

16. Choose the female chemical responsible for thickening the endometrium.
    a. Estrogen
    b. FSH
    c. TSH
    d. Progesterone

17. A sharp rise in LH, known as "LH surge," is responsible for:
    a. endometrial sloughing
    b. corpus luteal progression
    c. ripening of the Graafian follicle
    d. embryo maturation

18. Theca cells begin secreting estrogen:
    a. in utero
    b. at puberty
    c. at birth
    d. at ovulation

19. The number of oocytes in each ovary at puberty is approximately:
    a. one million
    b. 400
    c. 300,000
    d. one per month

20. Polymenorrheic is:
    a. a menstrual cycle length that is less than 21 days
    b. menstrual cycle length that is longer than 35 days
    c. heavy menstrual bleeding
    d. painful menstruation

21. Changes in endometrial thickness are not associated with:
    a. hyperplasia
    b. endometrial polyps
    c. carcinoma
    d. homogenous echotexture

22. Ovarian measurements are determined:
    a. on views in one plane and three dimensions: length, width, and depth
    b. on views in two orthogonal planes and three dimensions: length, width, and depth
    c. on views in one plane and two dimensions: length and depth
    d. on views in two orthogonal planes and two dimensions: length and width

23. What phase of the menstrual cycle do follicles become dominant?
    a. Luteal
    b. Early follicular
    c. Mid to late proliferative
    d. Late follicular

24. During the late proliferative phase, the endometrium thickens to approximately:
    a. 3 to 5 mm
    b. 9 to 12 mm
    c. 5 to 11 mm
    d. 7 to 9 mm

25. The triple line (three line sign) indicates the _____ stage.
    a. late proliferative
    b. late luteal
    c. early secretory
    d. mid-follicular

26. Amenorrhea is:
    a. heavy menstruation
    b. light menstruation
    c. painful menstruation
    d. menstrual cessation

27. Ultrasound is ordered in the postmenopausal patient most often for:
    a. pelvic pain
    b. vaginal bleeding
    c. abnormal lab values
    d. vaginal mucosal wrinkles

28. A thin layer separates the basal layer and the inner functional layer. The thin layer is:
    a. echogenic
    b. poorly defined
    c. 4- to 5-mm thick
    d. part of meiotic division

29. A 9- to 14-mm endometrium in the secretory phase appears:
    a. hypoechoic to the myometrium
    b. vascular
    c. echogenic with diffuse edematous and cystic collections
    d. echogenic with posterior enhancement

Fill-in-the-Blank

1. A female baby is born with approximately _____ oocytes in each ovary.

2. The uterus, fallopian tubes, two _____, cervix, _____, and the mammary glands make up the female reproductive internal organs.

3. The three uterine anatomical sections are _____, _____, and _____.

4. The two fallopian tubes are also known as _____ or _____.

5. Fimbriae sweep the _____ into the lumen of the fallopian tube.

6. The _____ ligament attaches to the uterus at the level of the cervix and from the superior part of the vagina to the lateral walls of the pelvis.

7. Located in the diencephalon, is the hypothalamus, which is positioned in the human _____.

8. The hypothalamus secretes hormones that stimulate and suppress the release of hormones in the _____ gland.

9. A female with abnormally light menstruation is diagnosed with _____.

10. Follicles house _____.

11. Ovaries function as _____ and endocrine glands.

12. Menstrual cycles can range from _____ to _____ days in adults and _____ to _____ in teens.

13. FSH is primarily responsible for promoting _____ development within the ovary.

14. LH is necessary for growth of _____ follicles and ovulation of the dominant follicle.

15. Endometrial maturation is caused by the hormone _____.

16. If fertilized egg implantation does not occur, the levels of _____ and _____ decrease, causing sloughing of the endometrium.

17. Two layers surround a developing follicle: _____ and _____.

18. _____ stimulates the endometrium to thicken before ovulation.

19. The three phases of the ovarian cycle are _____, _____, and _____.

20. Meiotic arrest of primary oocytes occurs until _____.

21. The endometrium should be measured on the _____ image, to include the anterior and posterior portions of the _____ endometrium.

22. Two layers of endometrium are shed during menses, _____ and _____.

23. When menstrual bleeding stops, the _____ phase begins.

24. Ultrasound imaging during the secretory phase demonstrates a uniformly _____ endometrium.

25. The most common hormonal disorder among reproductive age women is _____.

26. HRT is _____.

27. Changes in endometrial thickness can be associated with endometrial _____, _____, and _____.

Short Answer

1. A 72-year-old patient presented to her doctor complaining of one episode of spotting (light vaginal bleeding). Her physical examination was normal. Laboratory tests were ordered, as was a pelvic ultrasound to image female organs as well as the endometrium. Describe a normal postmenopausal endometrium.

2. What are expected endometrial measurements of a uterus in the menstrual phase, proliferative phase, and secretory phase?

3. Name a structure that releases progesterone during pregnancy. Explain the function of progesterone during pregnancy.

IMAGE EVALUATION/PATHOLOGY

Review the images and answer the following questions.

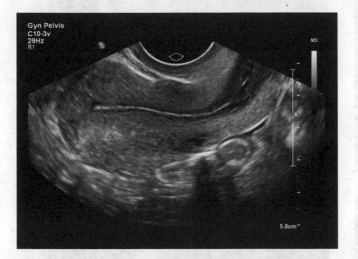

1. Identify the structure and the view. What phase is it?

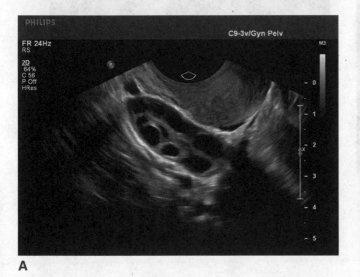

A

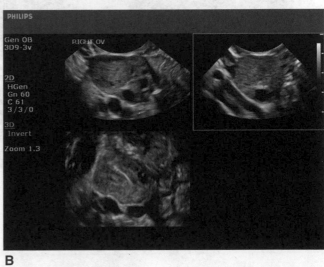

B

2. Name the structure in image A. What type of imaging produced image B?

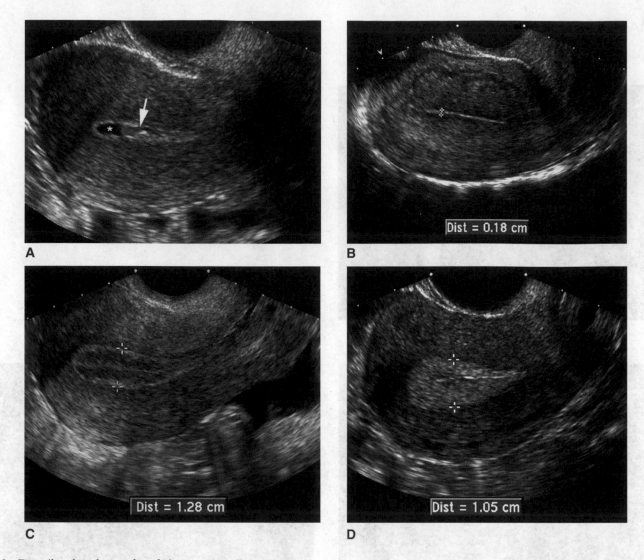

3. Describe the phase of each image, A to D.

CHAPTER 9

Normal Anatomy of the Female Pelvis

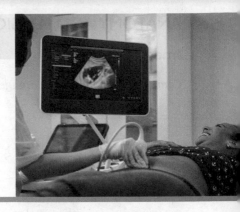

REVIEW OF GLOSSARY TERMS

Matching

Match the key terms with their definitions.

KEY TERMS

1. _____ pouch of Douglas

2. _____ corpora albicantia

3. _____ true pelvis

4. _____ follicular atresia

5. _____ serosa

6. _____ iliopsoas muscle

7. _____ linea terminalis

8. _____ anterior cul-de-sac

9. _____ hypertrophy

10. _____ fundus

11. _____ space of Retzius

12. _____ contralateral

13. _____ orthogonal

14. _____ iliopectineal line

15. _____ false pelvis

16. _____ ipsilateral

17. _____ follicle-stimulating hormone (FSH)

DEFINITIONS

a. Aka vesicouterine recess. Potential space between the uterus and urinary bladder
b. On the opposite side
c. Fibrous tissue that replaces the corpus luteum
d. Aka greater or major pelvis. Area superior to and anterior to the pelvic brim
e. Hormone that stimulates growth and maturation of the ovarian Graafian follicle. The anterior pituitary gland secretes the hormone.
f. Degeneration and reabsorption of the follicle before maturity
g. Latin anatomical term referring to the portion of an organ opposite from its opening
h. Aka pelvic brim or linea terminalis. Inner surface of the pubic and ilium bones contains a bony ridge that serves as the line dividing the true and false pelvis.
i. Increase in size
j. On the same side
k. Aka innominate line. Line drawn from the pubic crest to the arcuate line dividing the true and false pelvis
l. At right angles (perpendicular)
m. Aka posterior cul-de-sac or the rectouterine recess. Potential space between the rectum and uterus
n. Serous membrane enclosing an organ that often excretes lubricating serous fluid
o. Aka properitoneal space. Space between pubic symphysis and urinary bladder
p. Aka lesser or minor pelvis. Portion of the pelvic cavity inferior and posterior to the pelvic brim
q. Combination of the psoas major, psoas minor, and iliacus muscles

ANATOMY AND PHYSIOLOGY REVIEW

Image Labeling

Complete the labels in the images that follow.

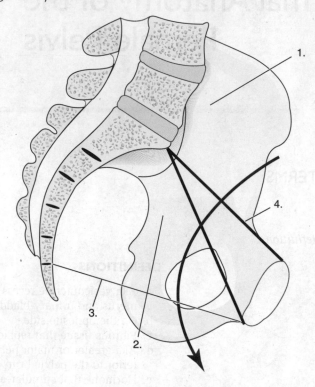

Pelvis anatomy

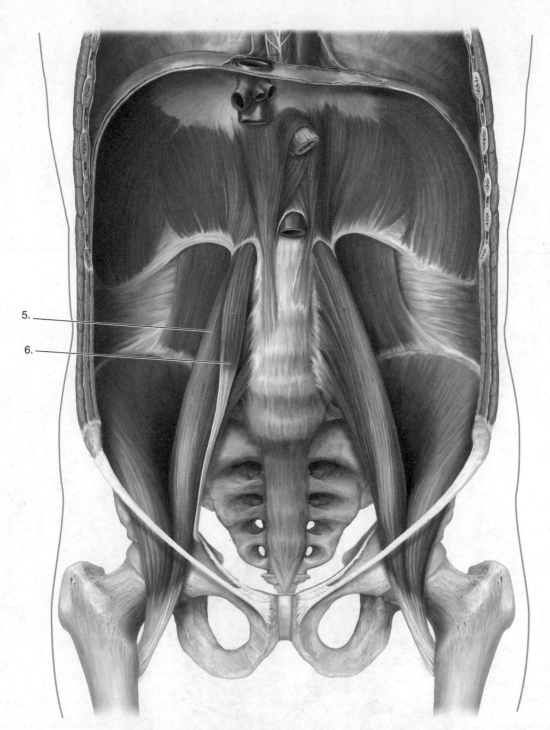

5.

6.

Posterior body wall and false pelvis muscles

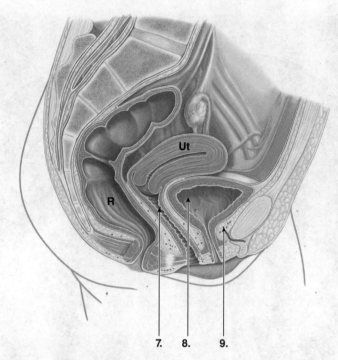

Midline sagittal female pelvis

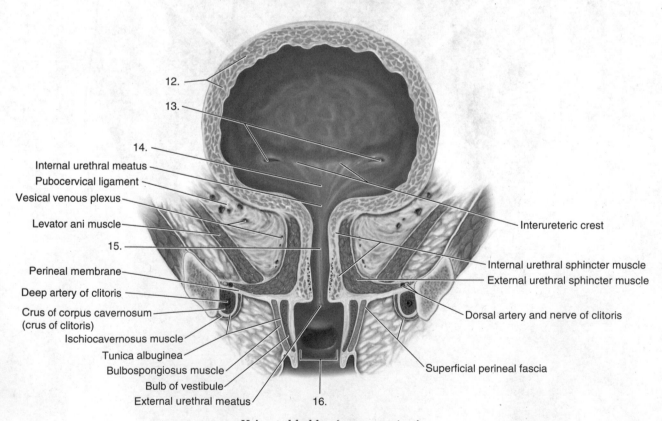

Urinary bladder (cutaway view)

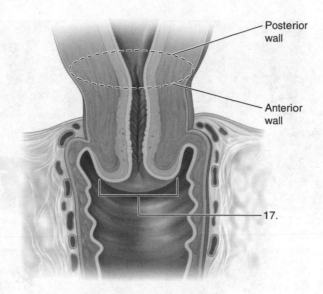

Posterior
wall

Anterior
wall

17.

Uterine vaginal relationship

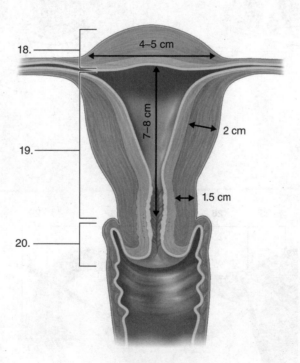

18.

4–5 cm

7–8 cm

2 cm

1.5 cm

19.

20.

Uterine sections

21.

22.

23.

24.

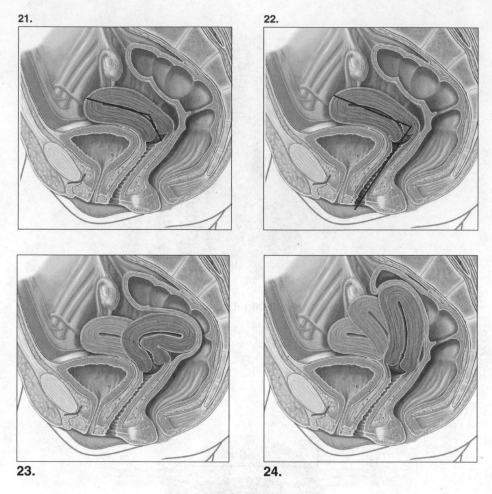

Uterine positions

25   26   27   28   29

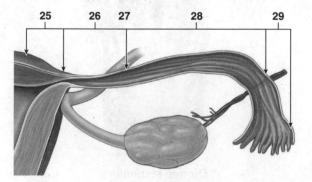

Fallopian tube regions

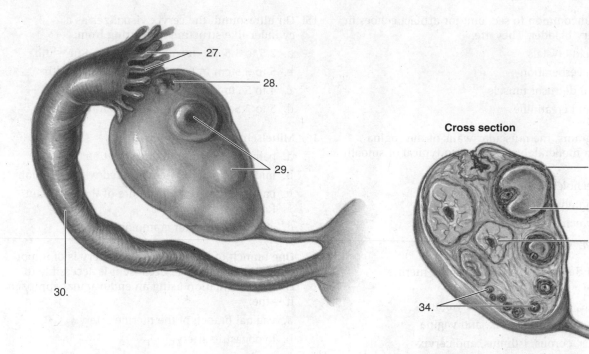

Ovary/fallopian tube, cross-section ovary

CHAPTER REVIEW

Multiple Choice

Complete each question by circling the best answer.

1. Choose the sonographic method that uses higher frequency transducers and markedly increases resolution of most pelvic structures?
   a. EVS
   b. Complimentary
   c. TAS general abdomen, obstetric, and gynecologic
   d. TAS deep abdomen, obstetric, and gynecologic

2. Choose the normal anatomic structure that EV imaging can easily identify.
   a. Vaginal fornices
   b. Sigmoid
   c. Ovaries
   d. Uterine serosa

3. What bones comprise the pelvic skeleton?
   a. Coccyx, sacrum, two innominate bones
   b. Sacrum, ischium, coccyx, ilium
   c. Pubic symphysis, sacrum, coccyx
   d. Two innominate bones, ilium, ischium

4. The rectus muscle is seen mostly in the lower abdomen in a(n):
   a. cylindrical shape
   b. hook with bulbous medial limb
   c. ovoid shape
   d. tubular shape

5. The cross-sectional shape of the iliopsoas muscle appears on ultrasound as:
   a. ovoid
   b. hook with bulbous medial limb
   c. hyperechoic coursing anteriorly
   d. cylindrical

6. The space of Retzius (preperitoneal space) is located:
   a. in the superior pelvis
   b. in the rectouterine recess
   c. fundally on the myometrium
   d. between the urinary bladder and symphysis pubis

7. It is not uncommon to see anterior artifact echoes in the urinary bladder. They are:
   a. uric acid crystals
   b. wall reverberation
   c. imaged detrusor muscle
   d. urea and creatinine

8. On sonograms, the muscular walls of the vagina produce a moderately ____ pattern typical of smooth muscle.
   a. hypoechoic
   b. moderately echogenic
   c. highly echogenic
   d. heterogeneous

9. Which of the following describes the uterine segments?
   a. Fundus, corpus, cervix, and vagina
   b. Corpus, isthmus, cervix, and vagina
   c. Fundus, corpus, isthmus, and cervix
   d. Fundus, interstitial, isthmus, and corpus

10. What is the largest portion of the uterus?
    a. Fundus
    b. Corpus
    c. Isthmus
    d. Cervix

11. The uterine layer not seen with ultrasound is:
    a. serosal (perimetrium)
    b. myometrial
    c. endometrial
    d. muscular

12. A uterus in a female infant would:
    a. appear cylindrical
    b. appear pear shape
    c. appear globular
    d. nonvisualize

13. Cysts of the cervix are caused by occluded cervical glands and known as:
    a. Gartner duct cyst
    b. dermoid cysts
    c. Nabothian cysts
    d. corpus luteum cysts

14. The length of the adult nulliparous uterus is approximately:
    a. 10 cm
    b. 2.5 cm
    c. 4 cm
    d. 8 cm

15. On ultrasound, the cervix visualizes as a cylinder-like structure measuring from:
    a. 2.5 to 3.5 cm in length and 2.5 cm in width
    b. 5 to 6.5 cm in length and 2.5 cm in width
    c. 4 to 5 cm in length and 3 cm in width
    d. 5 to 7.5 mm in length and 2.5 mm in width

16. Mittelschmerz is:
    a. pain associated with menstruation
    b. mid-cycle pain often associated with ovulation
    c. pain associated with rupture of the dominant follicle
    d. a medical term for cramping

17. One branch of the internal iliac artery is of importance to sonographers because it is accessible to Doppler evaluation using an endovaginal approach. It is the:
    a. vaginal branch of the uterine artery
    b. hypogastric artery
    c. uterine artery
    d. cervicouterine artery

18. Venous congestion appears as:
    a. thin-walled vessels
    b. dirty shadows
    c. pelvic varices
    d. short linear vessels

19. Echogenic ovarian foci may indicate the presence of all except:
    a. simple cysts
    b. malignancies
    c. endometriosis
    d. resolving hemorrhagic cyst

20. Fat or smooth muscles are more ____ than the skeletal muscles.
    a. superior
    b. linear
    c. hypoechoic
    d. echogenic

Fill-in-the-Blank

1. The pelvic organs are (1) the _____, (2) the _____ and _____, (3) the _____, _____, and _____, (4) the _____, and (5) the _____ and _____.

2. False pelvis anatomy includes _____ and _____.

3. Three functions of the female bony pelvis are _____, _____, and _____.

4. The urinary bladder lies between the _____ and the _____.

5. The urinary bladder is composed of _____ layers.

6. Only _____ of the many thousands of follicles that persist into adult life will actually progress through development and ovulation.

7. A partially filled bladder demonstrates its walls as _____, whereas a distended bladder demonstrates _____ walls.

8. _____ can be seen with color Doppler or high gain in gray-scale imaging when the ureteral valve opens with a bolus of urine to the bladder.

9. Bowel may be mistaken for a pelvic _____.

10. _____ and _____ make up the external genitalia.

11. Sonography also allows imaging of the female _____, _____, and urethra via transperitoneal ultrasound.

12. The posterior wall of the vagina is _____ than the anterior wall. The superior end of the vagina attaches to the _____.

13. The _____ is divided into sections called intramural, isthmic, and ampullary.

14. The ultrasound imaging method of choice for ovarian assessment is _____.

15. Echogenic ovarian foci (EOF), with or without shadowing, noted on an ovary may indicate the presence of _____.

16. The potential space between the rectum and uterus is _____.

17. The endometrium is a specialized mucosa that varies in _____, _____, and composition through the menstrual cycle.

18. A technique that aids in locating the fallopian tube is _____.

19. On both transabdominal and endovaginal ultrasound, the ovary may be identified by its characteristic "Swiss cheese" pattern of _____ follicles against the low-amplitude gray of the ovarian cortex.

20. To locate a "difficult" ovary, the examiner should _____ gain levels so that most of the echoes from the uterus and the parametrium disappear.

Short Answer

1. During pregnancy, the cervix provides a method of preventing bacteria to enter the uterus. Explain the process.

2. Explain the difference between the false pelvis and the true pelvis.

3. Which area, the space of Retzius or the pouch of Douglas, is more likely to collect free fluid?

4. A pelvic sonogram is revealing a solid hook-shaped mass on a thin posthysterectomy/oophorectomy (surgical removal of the uterus and ovaries) patient. Discuss the finding.

IMAGE EVALUATION/PATHOLOGY

Review the images and answer the following questions.

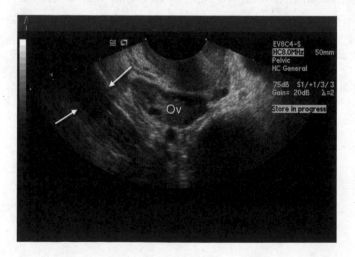

1. Name the structures the white arrows are directed toward.

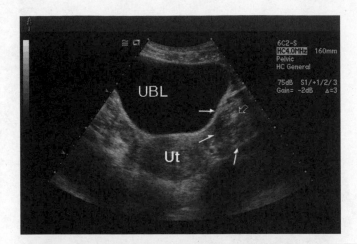

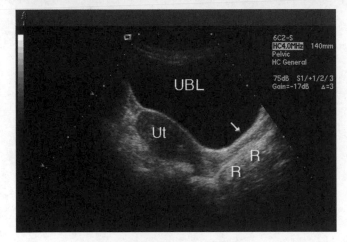

2. Name the structure the three white arrows are positioned around.

3. Name the structure the open arrow is pointing toward.

4. Name the structure the arrow is directed toward.

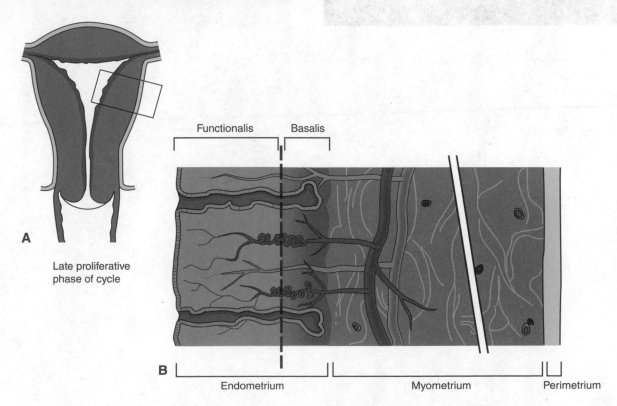

A

Late proliferative phase of cycle

B

Functionalis   Basalis

Endometrium   Myometrium   Perimetrium

5. Why is color flow seen in the image?

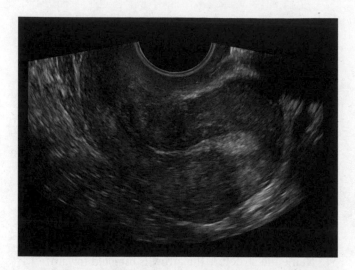

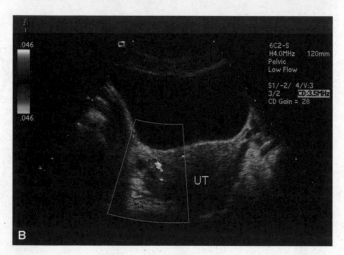

6. Explain the uterine position and scan orientation. *UT*, uterus; *B*, bowel.

7. Why is color seen at the lateral margin of the uterus?

CHAPTER 10

Doppler Evaluation of the Pelvis

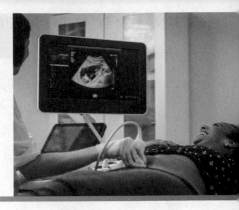

REVIEW OF GLOSSARY TERMS

Matching

Match the key terms with their definitions.

KEY TERMS

1. _____ pulsatility index

2. _____ ovarian vessels

3. _____ arteriovenous malformation

4. _____ impedance indices

5. _____ uterine artery

6. _____ S/D ratio

7. _____ Pourcelot resistive index

8. _____ adnexa

9. _____ secretory phase

10. _____ proliferative phase early

11. _____ arcuate vessels

12. _____ angiogenesis

13. _____ proliferative phase late

14. _____ resistive index

15. _____ specular reflectors

DEFINITIONS

a. When the sound wave encounters a distinct surface that is larger than the wavelength of the ultrasound beam

b. Physiologic process involving the growth of new blood cells from preexisting vessels

c. Small vascular structures found along the periphery of the uterus

d. Measurements used to compare the resistance of a medium to the propagation of flow

e. A sonographic indicator of an organ to perfusion. Calculated from the peak systolic velocity and the end-diastolic velocity of blood flow

f. Doppler measurement calculated by the value of the highest systolic peak minus the value of the highest diastolic peak divided by the highest systolic peak

g. Days 5 to 9 of the menstrual cycle

h. Days 10 to 14 of the menstrual cycle

i. Doppler measurement that uses peak systole minus peak diastole divided by the mean

j. Difference between peak systolic value and end-diastolic values of a vessel

k. Days 15 to 28 of the menstrual cycle

l. Main vessel carrying oxygenated blood toward the uterus

m. Abnormal connection between veins and arteries

n. Anatomical parts added, attached, or adjunct to another or others

o. Blood vessels that supply oxygenated blood to and drain deoxygenated blood away from the ovaries

ANATOMY AND PHYSIOLOGY REVIEW

Image Labeling

Complete the labels in the images that follow.

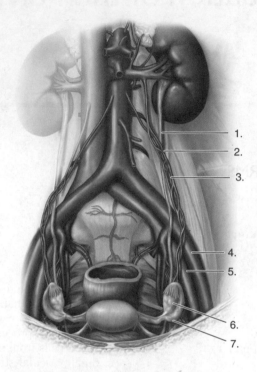

1. _____
2. _____
3. _____

4. _____
5. _____

6. _____
7. _____

Pelvic structures and vessels

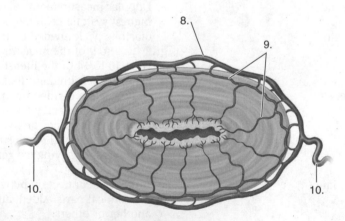

8. _____
9. _____

10. _____   10. _____

Diagram of arteries on a transverse uterus

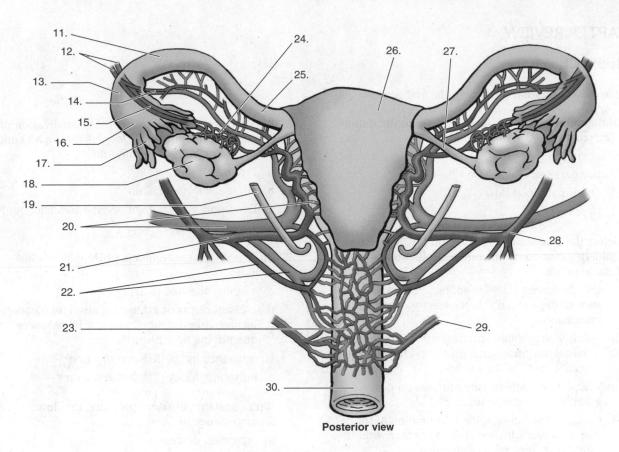

11.
12.
13.
14.
15.
16.
17.
18.
19.
20.
21.
22.
23.

24.
25.
26.
27.

28.

29.

30.

Posterior view

Uterine, vaginal, and ovarian blood supply

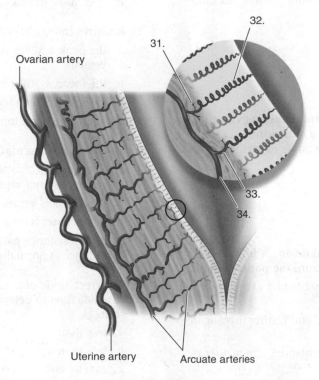

Ovarian artery

31.
32.
33.
34.

Uterine artery

Arcuate arteries

Arcuate arteries

CHAPTER REVIEW

Multiple Choice

Complete each question by circling the best answer.

1. Malignant tumors, benign tumors, and inflammatory conditions are not related to:
   a. angiogenesis
   b. normal physiologic blood flow
   c. abnormal blood flow
   d. hypoxia

2. Select the true statement regarding ACR practice guidelines for an ultrasound examination of the female pelvis:
   a. Use the lowest possible sonographic exposure settings to gain the necessary diagnostic information.
   b. Identify all relevant structures through transabdominal or transvaginal imaging, knowing that in few cases both will be needed.
   c. High-quality patient care requires no demographic documentation.
   d. Conduct the sonographic examination of the female pelvis with a real-time scanner without transducer frequency adjustment.

3. Choose the most appropriate transducer frequency for a transabdominal pelvic sonogram when more depth penetration is needed.
   a. 2.5 MHz
   b. 5.0 MHz
   c. 7.5 MHz
   d. 12 MHz

4. A full urinary bladder enhances uterine visualization, but frequently causes a suboptimal _____ Doppler exam owing to the angle of incidence.
   a. arcuate artery
   b. spiral artery
   c. radial artery
   d. uterine artery

5. If a cystic mass is suspected during a full bladder pelvic ultrasound examination, the patient should:
   a. partially void the urinary bladder and further investigate the pelvis
   b. void the urinary bladder and further investigate the pelvis
   c. fully distend the urinary bladder and further investigate the pelvis
   d. complete the examination under the current conditions

6. Which position provides the best visualization of free fluid in the pouch of Douglas during an endovaginal ultrasound examination?
   a. Prone
   b. Supine with vertical tilt
   c. Lithotomy with a slight reverse Trendelenburg
   d. Trendelenburg

7. Quantitative measurements of Doppler studies include:
   a. systolic/diastolic (S/D) ratios
   b. measurements of estimating absolute blood velocities, assessment of vascular impedances, and quantifying flow disturbances
   c. resistance index (RI) interrogation
   d. pulsatility index (PI) flow resistance

8. With constant perfusion pressure, the flow _____ as the impedance to flow _____.
   a. increases, decreases
   b. increases, increases
   c. remains constant, increases
   d. decreases, increases

9. Resistive index (RI) calculates:
   a. the peak systolic velocity to the end-diastolic velocity
   b. the mean systolic and diastolic ratio
   c. vascular impedance
   d. angle of insonation

10. Suspicion for vascular occlusion occurs when a:
    a. low resistance pattern is detected in a normally high resistance region
    b. waveform is erratic
    c. biphasic waveform is detected
    d. high resistance pattern is detected where low resistance is normally seen

11. A correct angle of _____ is required when analyzing vascular flow to determine its velocity by a Doppler shift.
    a. less than 60°
    b. less than 45°
    c. exactly 60°
    d. more than 90°

12. Normal arterial flow is seen as:
    a. recurring laminar flow with minimal sidewall turbulence
    b. alternating diastolic and systolic uptake
    c. alternating quick uptake systolic peak followed by a lower diastolic flow
    d. reduced peak systolic over diastolic

13. What is laminar flow?
    a. Blood velocity traveling the highest near the tunica intima (internal vessel wall)
    b. Uniform velocity through the vessel lumen
    c. Irregular flow because of vessel stricture
    d. Blood velocity traveling highest in the mid vessel

14. Name the vessel (appearing as a tubular structure) often seen sonographically in the outer uterine myometrium.
    a. Radial artery
    b. Arcuate artery
    c. Uterine artery
    d. Spiral artery

15. The functional layer of the endometrium is supplied blood by the:
    a. radial artery
    b. radial and spiral arteries
    c. arcuate and spiral arteries
    d. spiral artery

16. An arteriovenous malformation (AVM):
    a. is commonly seen in the cervix
    b. mostly involves the uterine endometrium
    c. is typically acquired through surgery or trauma
    d. is hyperechoic and well circumscribed

17. Choose a statement that is not related to pelvic congestion.
    a. Frequently diagnosed in nulliparous women
    b. Vulvar, perineal, and lower extremity varices
    c. Chronic dull pelvic ache
    d. Worsens with prolonged standing or walking

18. The best description of classic ovarian torsion is:
    a. free pelvic fluid
    b. an oval structure with peripheral cysts measuring approximately 7 mm
    c. an ovary with hypervascular patterns
    d. an enlarged, edematous ovary with multiple small peripheral follicles and little or no vascular flow

19. Complex cysts of the pelvis are:
    a. malignant if seen with papillary cystic projections and free fluid
    b. benign if void of a thick septa and thick walls
    c. difficult to discriminate because benign and malignant characteristics can be similar
    d. diagnosed only with Doppler evaluation

20. Which statement is correct?
    a. Low resistance flow has a low end-diastolic and peak systolic velocity.
    b. High resistance flow has a low end-diastolic value with a high peak systolic value.
    c. High resistance flow has a high end-diastolic and low peak systolic velocity.
    d. Arteries always demonstrate high resistance flow whereas veins always demonstrate low resistance flow.

Fill-in-the-Blank

1. _____ ultrasound is a vital component in the evaluation of pelvic pathology and physiology.

2. Following a transvaginal examination, clean the transducer with a(n) _____ solution.

3. Two ultrasound examinations that complement each other are _____ and _____.

4. A sonographer must question every patient about _____ allergies.

5. The uterine artery tends to be _____ and travels in a spiral fashion on the lateral aspect of the uterus.

6. The ovarian vein diameter in nulliparous women is _____ mm and can be up to _____ mm in women who have had children.

7. High and low _____ are the two types of arterial Doppler flow analysis.

8. The presence of blood flow in a select area or vessel, at a known depth, with a sample volume describes _____ Doppler.

9. The acronym BART means _____.

10. The standard measurement used when displaying the spectral waveform is velocity, which is written as _____.

11. Color Doppler, which is a color _____, is based on the amount of the frequency shift and the _____ they are moving in relation to the transducer.

12. Power or energy Doppler displays movement, but without the attempt to obtain a _____ shift.

13. Doppler ultrasound has been utilized as a noninvasive technique to assess blood flow _____.

14. The ovarian artery anastomoses with the _____ artery at the uterine cornua.

15. Mid-luteal phase uterine arterial flow mean values in premenopausal patients are similar to that of _____ patients.

16. The ureters and _____ arteries follow an inferior track over the _____ muscle.

17. The ovarian veins travel differently in the left pelvis than the right pelvis. The left ovarian vein courses _____ and drains into the left _____ vein. The _____ receives the right ovarian vein blood flow.

18. Although the gold standard for diagnosing pelvic congestion was traditionally _____, sonographic assessment with a _____ maneuver technique gave ultrasound an advantage with diagnosing pelvic congestion.

19. During pregnancy, veins _____ to accommodate increased blood _____.

20. The early proliferative phase is day _____ of the menstrual cycle.

Short Answer

1. Although the uterine artery can be imaged along the lateral uterine body, in what location is it visualized the best and using what ultrasound method?

2. Discuss the finding of a periuterine vein measuring greater than 5 mm in a nongravid uterus.

3. An infertility patient being sonographically examined in the early follicular phase of her cycle demonstrates limited color and power Doppler flow of her ovaries. Explain this finding.

4. Describe the appearance of arterial and venous waveforms. List benefits of knowing arterial versus venous flow within or external to a structure.

5. Identify arteries of the uterus from the perimetrium to the endometrium.

IMAGE EVALUATION/PATHOLOGY

Review the images and answer the following questions.

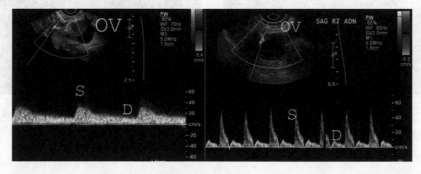

1. Describe the ovarian waveform of the left image and the right image. OV, ovary; S, systolic; D, diastolic.

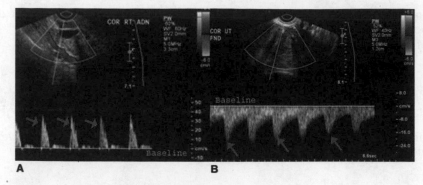

2. What direction is blood flowing in the left and right image.

   Hint: See baseline.

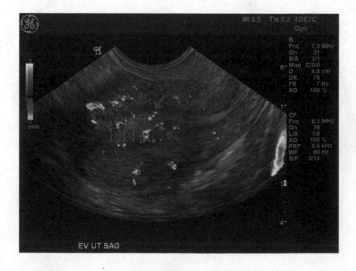

A

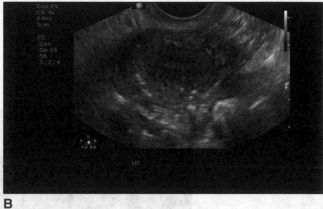

B

3. Explain the reason hyperechoic echoes are seen in this uterus.

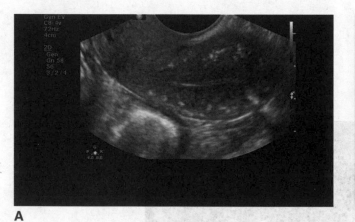

4. What vessels are the arrows directed toward in the sagittal endometrium?

Pediatric Pelvis

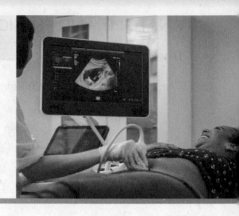

REVIEW OF GLOSSARY TERMS

Matching

Match the key terms with their definitions.

KEY TERMS

1. _____ diethylstilbestrol (DES)

2. _____ Turner syndrome

3. _____ gonadal dysgenesis

4. _____ adrenarche

5. _____ rhabdomyosarcoma

6. _____ hermaphrodite

7. _____ pseudohermaphrodite

8. _____ thelarche

9. _____ precocious puberty

10. _____ germ cell tumors

11. _____ Rokitansky nodule, aka dermoid plug

12. _____ pheochromocytoma

13. _____ Café au lait skin pigmentation

14. _____ ambiguous genitalia

DEFINITIONS

a. Increase in adrenal gland activity seen at the onset of puberty

b. Synthetic estrogen used from 1940 to 1971 to aid in pregnancy maintenance that resulted in T-shaped uterus in female children

c. Class of tumors that originate in either the egg or sperm

d. Loss of primordial germ cells in the gonads of an embryo

e. Having both male and female sexual characteristics

f. Vascular tumor of the adrenal gland

g. Early onset of puberty usually before 8 years of age

h. Individual with external genitalia of one sex and the internal organs of another sex

i. Malignancy derived from striated or skeletal muscle

j. Nodule projecting from a thickened cyst wall, usually ovarian in origin

k. Start of breast development at the onset of puberty

l. Genetic syndrome characterized by an X and O chromosome combination resulting in a female with premature ovarian failure and lack of puberty

m. Intersexual genitalia

n. Irregular flat spots of increased skin pigmentation

ANATOMY AND PHYSIOLOGY REVIEW

Image Labeling

Complete the labels in the images that follow.

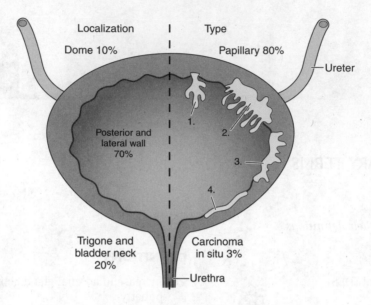

Urothelial neoplasms

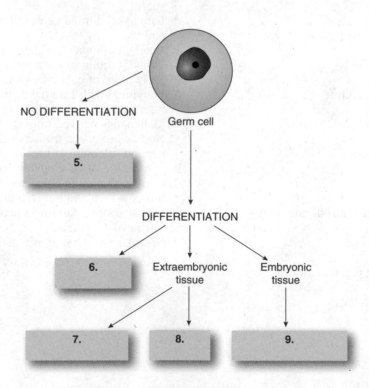

Classification of germ cell tumors of the ovary

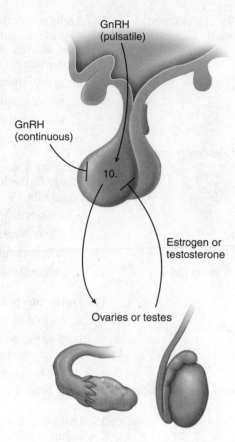

GnRH
(pulsatile)

GnRH
(continuous)

10.

Estrogen or
testosterone

Ovaries or testes

Gonadotropin-releasing hormone

CHAPTER REVIEW

Multiple Choice

Complete each question by circling the best answer.

1. An ineffective method of reducing adolescent anxiety prior to and during an ultrasound examination would be:

   a. singing songs and reciting nursery rhymes for younger adolescents

   b. allowing a bottle or pacifier for an infant

   c. providing a nurse chaperone

   d. permitting parents or loved ones to stay during the examination

2. When examining the pelvis of an infant or small child with ultrasound, which transducer is recommended?

   a. Phased array or curved linear in the range of 4 to 10 MHz

   b. Curved linear 5 MHz

   c. Linear 12 MHz

   d. Phased array or curved linear in the range of 1 to 5 MHz

3. Motion reduction on still images while imaging children can be attained by:

   a. giving instructions to hold their breath

   b. singing songs

   c. decreasing persistence

   d. using slightly more transducer pressure

4. Bladder filling for infants can usually be accomplished by feeding a bottle:

   a. 10 minutes prior to the sonographic examination

   b. 30 minutes prior to the sonographic examination

   c. 45 minutes prior to the sonographic examination

   d. 1 hour prior to the sonographic examination

5. A newborn female uterus is typically _____ shaped, whereas a 3-month-old uterus is usually _____ shaped.
    a. pear, cylindrical
    b. spade, pear
    c. pear, spade
    d. spade, tube

6. The best method to visualize an adolescent vagina is by:
    a. visual examination
    b. EVS (endovaginal sonography)
    c. TAS (transabdominal sonography)
    d. perineal imaging

7. Ovarian volume of a female under 5 years old is _____.
    a. 1 cm^3
    b. 1 cm^3 or less
    c. between 2 cm^3 and 3 cm^3
    d. 5 cm^3

8. Ovarian cysts measuring over 9 mm in the first year of life are known as:
    a. microcysts
    b. macrocysts
    c. simple cysts
    d. well-circumscribed cysts

9. The most common lower urinary tract tumor discovered in the pediatric community is:
    a. rhabdomyosarcoma
    b. medullary sarcoma
    c. chondrosarcoma
    d. fibrosarcoma

10. In the pediatric population, benign lesions of the lower urinary tract such as leiomyoma, fibroma, and hemangioma:
    a. occur in older adolescents more often than infants and young children
    b. occur in children associated with fetal alcohol syndrome
    c. are very uncommon
    d. may transition into cancer if untreated

11. The most common site of tumors in the pediatric female genital tract is the:
    a. uterus
    b. ovaries
    c. cervix
    d. vagina

12. An infection that can potentially affect the ovaries, uterus, and fallopian tubes and can cause tubo-ovarian abscess, endometritis, salpingitis, oophoritis, and/or pelvic peritonitis:
    a. hydrosalpinx
    b. pelvic inflammatory disease (PID)
    c. endometriosis
    d. urinary tract infection (UTI)

13. Rhabdomyosarcoma is the tumor found most commonly in the lower urinary tract of the pediatric population. This tumor usually originates from the:
    a. urinary bladder
    b. cervix/vagina
    c. fallopian tube
    d. genitourinary tract

14. Precocious puberty is:
    a. related to sexually active adolescents
    b. a secretion of the lining of ovarian cysts in adolescence
    c. the onset of puberty usually before 8 years of age
    d. is related to sexually abused pediatric patients

15. Large ovarian cysts are common in fetuses of mothers with:
    a. toxemia
    b. choriocarcinoma
    c. arrhenoblastoma
    d. granulosa theca

16. Select Turner syndrome characteristics.
    a. Stocky arms and legs, wide neck, genital underdevelopment
    b. Polydactyly, abnormal genitalia, omphalocele
    c. Deficient ovaries, dwarfism, amenorrhea, webbed neck
    d. Choroid plexus cyst, polyhydramnios, esophageal atresia

17. Ambiguous genitalia in neonates warrants sonography to exclude anomalies associated with:
    a. gonads, adrenal glands, kidneys
    b. internal and external genitalia, spleen, kidneys
    c. breast lumps, internal genitalia
    d. gonads, liver, pancreas, spleen

18. The most common ultrasound appearance of a rhabdomyosarcoma is described as:
    a. heterogenous with 2- to 4-mm calculi and irregular borders
    b. hypoechoic with well-defined walls measuring 1 mm
    c. homogenous with sharp thin borders
    d. homogenous with a muscle-like appearance

19. Gartner duct cysts:
    a. are located within the uterine myometrium and complex in appearance
    b. are located within the vaginal wall, have a simple cystic appearance, and are both single or multiple in number
    c. are located within the cervix and are hypoechoic solid structures
    d. are located within the vagina and are heterogeneous

20. Hematometrocolpos is:
    a. blood in the vagina
    b. blood in the cervix
    c. blood in the uterus
    d. blood in both the uterus and vagina

Fill-in-the-Blank

1. The method of ultrasound imaging that is close to the vagina and does not require the introduction of a transducer into the vagina is called _____.

2. High-resolution, real-time, and _____ are important imaging techniques for the lower abdominal and pelvic structures of infants, children, and adolescents.

3. In adolescent pelvic sonography, _____ may be required if bladder filling cannot be achieved by p.o. (by mouth) fluid intake.

4. Adult and pediatric ultrasound examinations are similar in scanning _____ and exam _____.

5. Transperineal ultrasound imaging delineates _____ pathology and imperforate _____.

6. The prepubertal uterus measures _____ cm long.

7. Ovarian cysts in birth to 2-year-olds usually relate to a higher level of _____ in the neonate.

8. When a tumor, such as a rhabdomyosarcoma, originates from the bladder or prostate, pediatric patients have symptoms of _____ and _____.

9. In the pediatric pelvis, pheochromocytoma is usually detected in the submucosal layer of the _____ wall of the bladder near the _____ or in the _____ of the bladder.

10. Ovarian tumors present with a variety of symptoms including _____, _____, and _____.

11. The most common tumor during the reproductive years is a _____.

12. Meig syndrome is the triad of _____, _____, and _____.

13. Dysgerminoma is the most common malignant pediatric _____ mass.

14. Serous tumor usually demonstrates _____ septa, solid elements, and are _____.

15. Ovarian cysts may cause ovarian _____ if they become large.

16. Gonadal dysgenesis patients may have _____ gonads.

17. Fluid in the vagina is _____ and blood in the vagina is _____.

18. Fluid in both the uterus and vagina is _____.

19. The sonographic appearance of hydrocolpos is a cystic, _____-shaped mass in the midline arising from the pelvis between the bladder and _____.

20. Clinical symptoms of ovarian torsion are _____, _____, _____, _____, and _____.

Short Answer

1. Internal gynecology examinations are usually not possible or desirable in young girls. Ultrasound can provide a painless and unobtrusive method to examine pelvic organs. List indications for a gynecologic ultrasound examination in a young female.

2. Ovarian torsion occurs mostly occurs in which pelvic adnexa.

3. Explain where rhabdomyosarcoma is usually discovered in the pediatric population. Describe the typical sonographic appearance.

4. A sexually active 14-year-old girl complaining of a "lump" in her mid-pelvis and mild sporadic pelvic pain for 2 weeks presented to her doctor and was found to have a midline low pelvic mass measuring approximately 10 cm long and 6 cm wide. There was no visual indication of vaginal bleeding. Her menses had been irregular since onset. State a possible diagnosis.

5. Explain the difference between hydrocolpos, hydrometra, hematometra, hematocolpos, hydrometrocolpos, and hematometrocolpos.

IMAGE EVALUATION/PATHOLOGY

Review the images and answer the following questions.

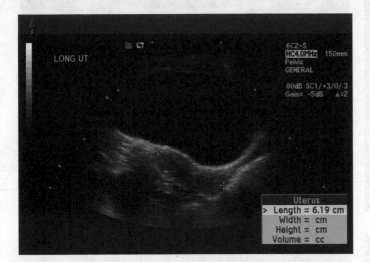

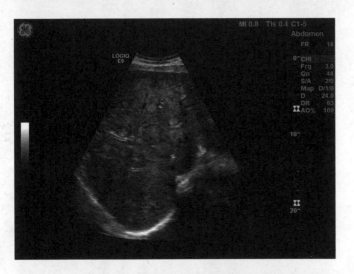

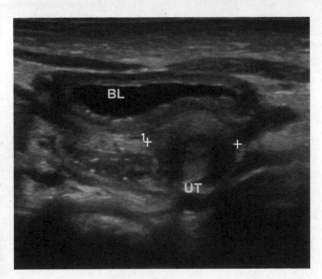

1. Identify the organ seen within the calipers.

2. Name the structure seen in the image.

3. Identify the organ seen in the transverse image within the calipers. BL, bladder; UT, uterus.

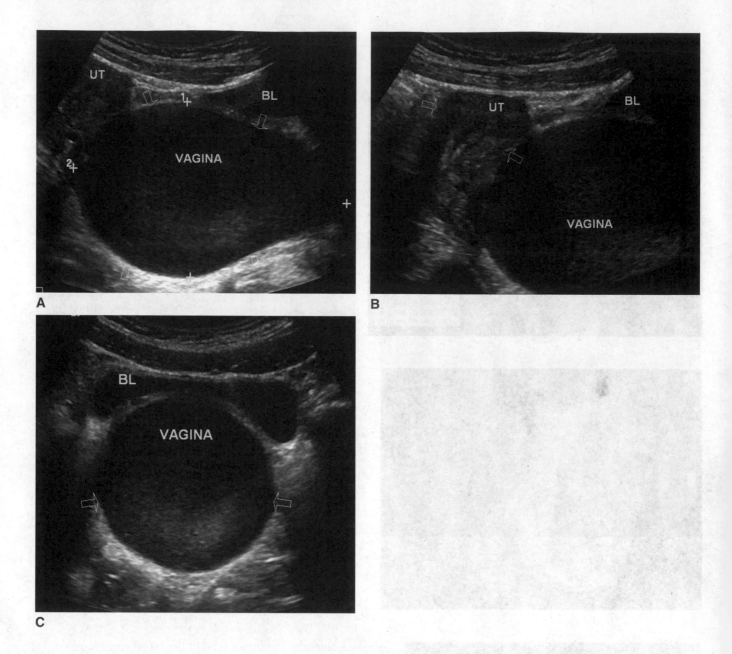

4. Diagnose the condition imaged in the three images. BL, bladder; UT, uterus.

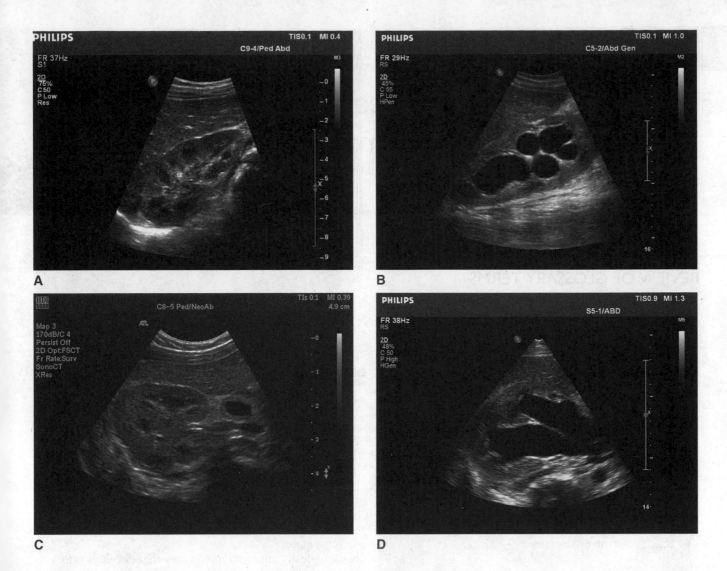

A

B

C

D

5. State the anatomy and condition of the organ in the four images.

CHAPTER 12

Benign Disease of the Female Pelvis

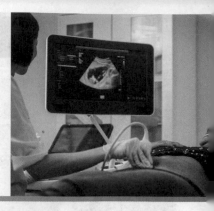

REVIEW OF GLOSSARY TERMS

Matching

Match the key terms with their definitions.

KEY TERMS

1. _____ adhesiolysis

2. _____ psammoma bodies

3. _____ endometrioma

4. _____ lysis

5. _____ hysteroscope

6. _____ uterine dehiscence

7. _____ electrosurgery

8. _____ oligomenorrhea

9. _____ hirsutism

10. _____ red degeneration

11. _____ hyperandrogenism

12. _____ omentum

13. _____ tamoxifen

14. _____ follicle-stimulating hormone (FSH)

15. _____ involute

16. _____ anovulation

17. _____ placenta previa

18. _____ hyperandrogenemia

DEFINITIONS

a. Surgical removal of adhesions (scar tissue)
b. Failure to ovulate
c. Inflammation of the bowel
d. Surgery performed with an electrical device such as an electrocautery
e. Blood-filled ovarian cyst resultant from endometriosis implants
f. Hormone produced by the anterior pituitary gland which stimulates growth of the Graafian follicle
g. Form of carcinoma that grows into the uterine musculature
h. Genetically abnormal pregnancy that develops into a grape-like mass within the uterus
i. Increased testosterone levels associated with PCOS
j. Excessive production/secretion of androgens
k. Reconstructive surgery of the uterus
l. Instrument allowing visualization of the uterus
m. Collapsing and rolling inward
n. Hormone produced by the anterior pituitary gland which stimulates ovulation
o. Breaking up of tissue
p. Abnormally heavy or prolonged menses
q. Infrequent menses
r. Infrequent ovulation
s. Peritoneal fold supporting the abdominal viscera
t. Growth of the placenta into the myometrium
u. Implantation of the placenta in the lower uterine segment or on the cervix
v. Microscopic collection of calcium associated with specific tumor types
w. Tissue that absorbs X-rays appearing white on the resulting radiograph
x. Hemorrhage into a leiomyoma that has outgrown its blood supply

19. _____ radiodense (radiopaque)

20. _____ hysteroplasty

21. _____ luteinizing hormone (LH)

22. _____ Crohn disease

23. _____ placenta accrete

24. _____ hydatidiform mole

25. _____ menorrhagia

26. _____ oligoanovulation

27. _____ chorioadenoma destruens

y. Antiestrogenic drug used to decrease the occurrence of certain estrogen-sensitive breast cancers
z. Partial separation of the myometrium at the location of uterine scar
aa. Excessive hair on a woman

ANATOMY AND PHYSIOLOGY REVIEW

Image Labeling

Complete the labels in the images that follow.

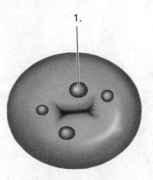

Cervical cyst

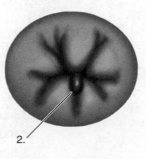

Cervical neoplasm

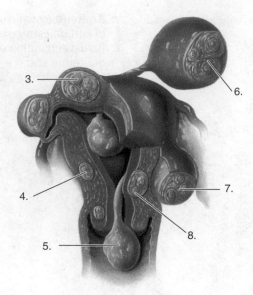

Leiomyoma locations

CHAPTER REVIEW

Multiple Choice

Complete each question by circling the best answer.

1. Select the cervical anomaly that does not cause bleeding.
   a. leiomyoma
   b. polyp
   c. Nabothian cyst
   d. hyperplasia

2. HSG is:
   a. hysterosalpingography
   b. hysteroscopic guidance
   c. hysterosonography
   d. hysteroplastic service guide

3. Uterine dehiscence is caused by:
   a. subserosal and intramural fibromas
   b. endometrial and cervical polyps
   c. multiparity
   d. uterine surgeries such as cesarean section (C/S)

4. Leiomyomas:
   a. occur in 50% to 60% of women of reproductive age
   b. are the most common tumor of the female pelvis
   c. usually occur after menopause
   d. are also known as myometra

5. Degenerative changes occur when myomas:
   a. become larger than 3 cm
   b. become painful
   c. outgrow their blood supply
   d. fibrotic menorrhagia occurs

6. Sonohysterography (SHSG):
   a. produces radiation to the patient
   b. may cause bleeding, intense pain, and provide ovarian contour information
   c. is performed in place of a myomectomy
   d. demonstrates myomatous extension onto the endometrium through visualizing filling defects

7. Imaging identification of a previous cesarean section (C/S) scar can be performed most effectively by:
   a. endovaginal sonography
   b. transabdominal sonography
   c. transperineal sonography
   d. hysteroscopy

8. Differentiating a pelvic mass from bowel may be done by:
   a. monitoring the suspect area for peristalsis
   b. noting fluid levels
   c. demonstrating gas bubble formation
   d. measurements

9. Lymphoceles, uromas, hematomas, and abscesses:
   a. are easily differentiated because each has unique attributes
   b. share sonographic characteristics of cystic structures with septations
   c. display similar laboratory results
   d. cause distinct symptoms

10. A fibromyoma located within the myometrium is labeled:
    a. subserosal/serosal
    b. pedunculated
    c. intramural
    d. submucosal

11. Anechoic or complex lesions of the superior antero-lateral vagina wall (adjacent to the cervix) are:
    a. Nabothian cysts
    b. fibroid cysts
    c. Bartholin gland cyst
    d. Gartner duct cyst

12. Select the sonographic criteria most likely not related to benign ovarian cysts.
    a. Lack of color flow within the cystic structure
    b. Increased posterior enhancement
    c. Homogeneously increased echogenicity
    d. Smooth posterior border

13. The "ring of fire" demonstrated peripherally when imaging a cyst with color or power Doppler is related to:
    a. theca lutein cysts
    b. corpus luteum cysts
    c. surface epithelial inclusion cysts
    d. hemorrhagic cysts

14. Sonographic findings in serous cystadenoma compared to mucinous cystadenoma are:
    a. generally similar, therefore, may be difficult to diagnose from imaging
    b. serous displays cystic fluid–fluid levels, mucinous appears cystic with projections from the cyst wall
    c. serous shows simple pinpoint echoes, mucinous shows thick walls
    d. serous demonstrates a hemorrhagic appearance, mucinous demonstrates multilocularity

15. Gonadoblastoma tumors may cause all of the following except:
    a. primary amenorrhea
    b. abscess
    c. abnormal genitalia
    d. virilization

16. Meigs syndrome presents as:
    a. enlarged ovaries demonstrating a "string of pearls" sign
    b. simple cysts usually measuring 7 to 10 cm
    c. ascites, pleural effusion, and an ovarian neoplasm
    d. thick-walled, irregular contoured cysts.

17. Select the description for ovarian remnant syndrome.
    a. Severe adhesions and endometriosis
    b. FSH/LH hyperstimulation
    c. Unilateral oophorectomy
    d. Bilateral salpingo-oophorectomy followed by restored function of remnant ovarian tissue

18. A posthysterectomy AP vaginal cuff should measure:
    a. 2.0×3.5 cm
    b. greater than 3.1 cm
    c. 4.2×2.0 cm
    d. less than 2.2 cm

19. A cystadenoma is a _____ tumor originating in glandular tissue.
    a. cervical
    b. malignant
    c. benign
    d. solid

20. Paraovarian cysts arise from the:
    a. adnexa
    b. ovarian epithelium
    c. ovarian stroma
    d. cervix

Fill-in-the-Blank

1. Excessive growth of the endometrium is a condition called _____.

2. The gold standard diagnostic procedure for the uterus and fallopian tubes is _____.

3. Asherman syndrome, which is _____ of the endometrium, is also known as _____.

4. A condition in which the uterine myometrium separates leaving an intact peritoneum is _____.

5. Uterine scarring caused by cesarean section occurs on the _____ of the _____ at the _____ of the _____.

6. Techniques that may help demonstrate myomas include _____, _____, and increase the output power because myomas tend to attenuate the sound beam.

7. _____ formation within the pelvis may be owing to an infectious process involving the tubes, ovaries, appendix, bowel, peritoneum, or bowel perforation.

8. The sonographic appearance of a lymphocele is a pocket of fluid with a well-defined _____ mass.

9. Leiomyomas are also called _____, _____, and _____.

10. Multiple large subserosal myomas may result in an _____ uterus with a _____ contour; large intramural and submucous myomas may distend the uterine _____ and distort the _____.

11. The normal appendix measures less than _____ from outer edge to outer edge.

12. If fallopian tubes are detected sonographically as tubular, tortuous, and fluid-filled, a diagnosis may be _____ or _____.

13. Functional or physiologic cysts of the ovary include _____, _____, _____, and _____.

14. Cysts greater than 10 cm in size have a greater potential to be _____ or invasive.

15. Ovarian torsion presents mostly on the _____ side and demonstrates _____ of blood flow.

16. Fibrothecomas demonstrate a _____ contour, _____, and _____.

17. _____ are fluid-filled masses caused by serous fluid collections between layers of peritoneum or adhesions.

18. Gonadoblastoma size ranges up to _____ cm. They demonstrate areas of _____.

19. Cysts measuring less than _____ cm in greatest diameter usually regress spontaneously.

20. Tumors containing teeth, hair, glandular tissues, and possibly neural or thyroid tissue are _____ or _____ tumors.

Short Answer

1. Define endometrial hyperplasia and explain its appearance on a sonographic image. List common reasons women develop endometrial hyperplasia.

2. Explain hysterosalpingography and the safest time to perform the examination.

3. A 48-year-old patient with known myomas has recently suffered increased vaginal bleeding during her menses. Why is it important to measure the myomas and detect their location?

4. A 33-year-old G3 P3 was delivered by C/S 1 month ago. Previous to the scheduled delivery, she had requested and consented to a tubal ligation that was performed immediately following the birth of her child. Over the last month, she has complained of tenderness in the left low pelvis. Ultrasound demonstrated a 3.8 × 4.3 × 3.8 cm hypoechoic left adnexal mass with internal debris adjacent to the uterus. CT followed and demonstrated a 4.0-cm loculated fluid collection in the same location. State a probable diagnosis. Describe symptoms that the patient may have.

5. Compare benign cystic teratoma to dermoid tumor.

IMAGE EVALUATION/PATHOLOGY

Review the images and answer the following questions.

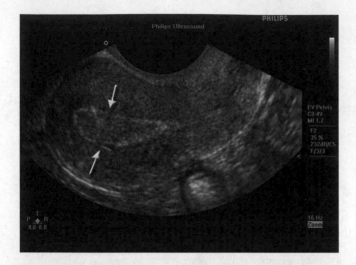

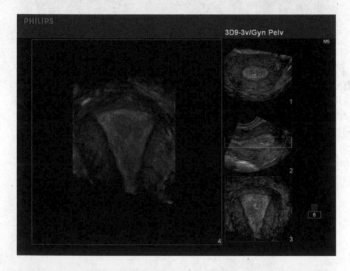

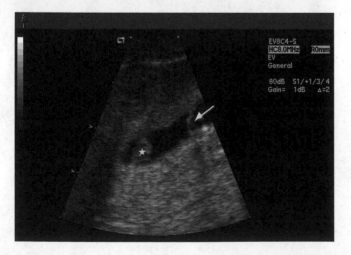

1. Name the anatomy. Identify the structure depicted by the two arrows. Name the method used to obtain the image.

2. How was this image collected? What is the structure demonstrated? Label the views adjacent to 1, 2, and 3.

3. A saline infusion sonohysterography (SIS) was performed on this sagittal uterus. Label the structure the arrow points toward, and the structure the star is placed on.

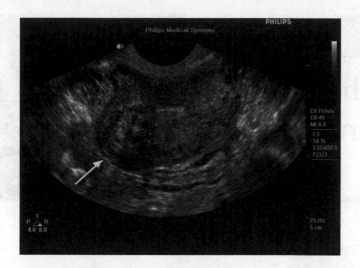

4. Define the structure the arrow points toward.

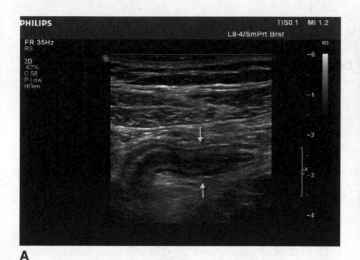

A

B

5. Define the anatomy. Explain the two images.

CHAPTER 13

Malignant Disease of the Uterus and Cervix

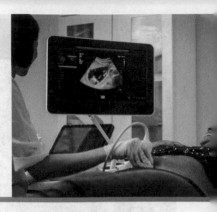

REVIEW OF GLOSSARY TERMS

Matching

Match the key terms with their definitions.

KEY TERMS

1. _____ pelvic inflammatory disease

2. _____ resistive index (RI)

3. _____ epithelioid trophoblastic tumor

4. _____ adenosis

5. _____ cervical stenosis

6. _____ leiomyosarcoma

7. _____ brachytherapy

8. _____ endometrial hyperplasia

9. _____ antineoplastic

10. _____ human papilloma virus (HPV)

11. _____ teratogenic

12. _____ polycystic ovarian syndrome

13. _____ methotrexate

14. _____ granulosa cell tumor

15. _____ androstenedione

16. _____ squamous cell carcinoma

17. _____ persistent trophoblastic neoplasia (PTN)

18. _____ human chorionic gonadotropin (hCG)

19. _____ choriocarcinoma

DEFINITIONS

a. Malignant tumor arising from any glandular organ

b. Any disease of a gland or of glandular tissue, especially the abnormal proliferation of the glandular tissue

c. Naturally occurring steroid hormone, accessible as a dietary supplement and believed to increase serum testosterone levels

d. Any substance that blocks or modifies the action of estrogen

e. Prevents the development, growth, or proliferation of malignant cells

f. Growth protruding from the epithelium of the cervix; may be broad based or pedunculated

g. Narrowing or obstruction or the cervical canal caused by an acquired condition

h. Metastatic type of persistent trophoblastic neoplasia that can result from any type of pregnancy but most often occurs with molar pregnancy

i. Malignant layer of cells that form in the endometrium; presents with abnormal thickening of the endometrial cavity and irregular bleeding in peri-menopausal and postmenopausal women

j. Condition that results from estrogen stimulation to the endometrium without the influence of progestin; frequent cause of bleeding especially in postmeno-pausal women

k. Pedunculated or sessile mass growing from the endometrium

l. Tumor that microscopically resembles endometrial tissue

m. Variant of placental-site trophoblastic tumor

n. Malignancy of the fallopian tube which is also linked to BRCA-1 and BRCA-2; adenocarcinoma is the most common histologic type

o. Rare earth metallic element possessing paramagnetic properties that are used in contrast media for magnetic resonance imaging (MRI)

20. _____ hydrops tubae profluens

21. _____ gadolinium

22. _____ endometrial carcinoma

23. _____ cervical polyp

24. _____ placental-site trophoblastic tumor (PSTT)

25. _____ leiomyoma

26. _____ Peutz-Jeghers syndrome

27. _____ salpingo-oophorectomy

28. _____ pulsatility index (PI)

29. _____ endometrial polyp

30. _____ Papanicolaou (pap) smear

31. _____ gestational trophoblastic neoplasia

32. _____ submucosal leiomyoma

33. _____ adenocarcinoma

34. _____ endometrioid

35. _____ fallopian tube carcinoma

36. _____ sonohysterography

37. _____ specificity

38. _____ metastases

39. _____ antiestrogen

40. _____ invasive mole

41. _____ radiation therapy

42. _____ polypoid

43. _____ sensitivity

44. _____ tamoxifen

p. Group of rare diseases in which abnormal trophoblast cells overtake pregnancy and propagated throughout the uterine cavity; these tumors arise from the placental chorionic villi after conception.

q. Estrogen secreting tumor that arises from granulosa cells. These tumors are part of the sex cord-gonadal stromal category and present as large, complex, ovarian masses.

r. Hormone produced by chorionic cells in the fetal part of the placenta and found in the urine and blood of pregnant women; elevated levels are found with GTN.

s. Virus that is transmitted through sexual contact and produces lesions on the mucous membranes; most common sexually transmitted infection and considered a causative factor in cervical carcinoma

t. Watery discharge sometimes present with fallopian tube carcinoma

u. Form of persistent gestational trophoblastic neoplasia typically deriving from a hydatidiform mole that invades into the myometrium

v. Benign tumor composed of smooth muscle cells and fibrous connective tissue that occurs in the uterus

w. Malignant uterine tumor that is composed of smooth muscle cells and fibrous connective tissue; sonographically appears like benign leiomyoma

x. Process by which cancer spreads from a primary source to distant locations in the body

y. Drug that inhibits cellular reproduction; used primarily in the treatment of psoriasis, various malignant neoplastic diseases, and as an immunosuppressive agent

z. Cytologic study (developed by George Nicholas Papanicolaou) used to detect cancer in cells that an organ has shed; used most often in the diagnosis and prevention of cervical cancer and also valuable in the detection of pleural or peritoneal malignancies

aa. Infection of the uterus, fallopian tubes, and adjacent pelvic structures; usually caused by an ascending infection in which disease-producing germs spread from the vagina and cervix to the upper portions of the female reproductive tract

bb. Malignant end of the GTN spectrum. This group of life-threatening diseases persists most often from a molar pregnancy.

cc. Inherited disorder characterized by the presence of polyps of the small intestine and melanin pigmentation of the lips, mucosa, fingers, and toes; anemia from the intestinal polyp is common.

dd. Type of PTN that usually occurs several years after a normal term pregnancy

ee. Complex disorder involving infrequent, irregular menstrual cycles and often excess male hormone (androgen) levels

ff. Growth similar to a polyp

gg. Calculation of Doppler measurements of systolic and diastolic velocities during a specified cardiac cycle; like the resistive index, it is used to assess the resistance in a pulsatile vascular system.

hh. Treatment technique that uses high doses of radiation to kill cancer cells and shrink tumors; deters the proliferation of malignant cells by decreasing mitosis or by impairing DNA synthesis

ii. Calculated flow parameter in ultrasound used to assess the resistance in a pulsatile vascular system

jj. (True negative rate) measures the proportion of those individuals who do not have the condition and who are correctly identified as not having the condition

kk. Injection of sterile saline into the endometrial canal under ultrasound guidance; this procedure allows for good visualization of the endometrial borders to rule out pathology.

ll. Slow-growing malignant tumor composed of squamous epithelium; most common type of cervical cancer

mm. Type of leiomyoma that deforms the endometrial cavity and can cause heavy or irregular menses

nn. Nonsteroidal antiestrogen compound that is currently the most widely prescribed drug for the treatment of breast cancer

oo. Causing congenital anomalies or birth defects

pp. (True positive rate) measures the portion of those individuals having some condition and who are correctly identified as having the condition

qq. Surgical removal of the fallopian tubes and ovaries

rr. Procedure that involves placing radioactive material inside the body to treat

CHAPTER REVIEW

Multiple Choice

Complete each question by circling the best answer.

1. Select the factor most unlikely to contribute to endometrial cancer.
   a. Obesity, particularly those more than 50 pounds overweight
   b. Unopposed estrogen such as hormone replacement therapy
   c. Thin habitus
   d. Polycystic ovarian syndrome

2. Tamoxifen therapy is known to increase the risk of all except:
   a. endometrial hyperplasia.
   b. polyps.
   c. myomas.
   d. endometrial cancer.

3. Endometrial cancer typically presents as:
   a. uterine bleeding.
   b. bloating.
   c. urinary frequency.
   d. persistent indigestion and constipation.

4. Select the least helpful imaging method for providing accurate diagnostic tumor angiogenesis information.
   a. EV
   b. TA
   c. 3D
   d. Color and pulsed Doppler

5. Which condition will not cause the endometrium to appear thickened?
   a. Myomas
   b. Menstrual phase
   c. Endometrial hyperplasia
   d. Endometrial cancer

6. Leiomyosarcomas:
   a. are slow growing.
   b. are heterogeneous.
   c. do not display blood flow.
   d. are never palpable.

7. Fallopian tube carcinoma is an aggressive tumor that demonstrates all except a:
   a. sausage-shaped mass in the adnexa.
   b. cystic mural nodular mass lateral to the uterus.
   c. thickened endometrium.
   d. hydrosalpinx.

8. A frequent suspicious characteristic of fallopian tube carcinoma is:
   a. pelvic ascites.
   b. bilateral groin pain.
   c. circumscribed simple cystic adnexal collection less than 0.5 cm.
   d. decreased CA-125.

9. Fallopian tube carcinoma may cause suspicious characteristics of all except:
   a. intrauterine fluid.
   b. tumor lakes.
   c. a trilaminar homogeneous endometrium.
   d. hydrosalpinx.

10. Infection by HPV is the largest cause of:
    a. fallopian tube carcinoma.
    b. ovarian adenocarcinoma.
    c. primary uterine carcinoma.
    d. cervical carcinoma.

11. Exposure to DES (diethylstilbestrol) in utero causes an increased incidence of adenocarcinoma of the:
    a. cervix and ovary.
    b. cervix and vagina.
    c. uterus and fallopian tube.
    d. fallopian tube and ovary.

12. Cervical stenosis caused by cervical cancer may cause:
    a. cogwheel appearance of an adnexa lesion.
    b. copious watery vaginal discharge.
    c. hematometra.
    d. arteriovenous shunts.

13. Select the imaging modality that is least helpful with diagnosing fallopian tube neoplasia.
    a. MRI
    b. CT
    c. EV US
    d. Transabdominal ultrasound

14. Choose the imaging modality that has excellent soft-tissue contrast resolution and is therefore significantly valuable in the assessment of the size of the tumor, the depth of the cervical cancer invasion.
    a. Ultrasound
    b. CT
    c. MRI
    d. Radiography

15. Select the phrase used to describe a group of uterine neoplasms that occur as a complication of pregnancy.
    a. Gestational trophoblastic neoplasia (GTN)
    b. Placental-site trophoblastic tumor (PSTT)
    c. Choriocarcinoma tumors (CT)
    d. Malignant gestational neoplasia (MGN)

16. Gestational trophoblastic neoplasia:
    a. increases Nabothian cysts.
    b. demonstrates a bulky cervical appearance.
    c. can occur as a complication of ectopic pregnancy.
    d. can occur as a complication of all pregnancies.

17. Invasive mole is a form of hydatidiform mole that invades the:
    a. myometrium.
    b. fallopian tube(s).
    c. perimetrium.
    d. vagina.

18. Although clinical signs for endometrial cancer and leiomyosarcomas are nonspecific, most present with:
    a. trace amounts of free fluid.
    b. uterine bleeding and pain.
    c. irregular bowel habits.
    d. hydronephrosis.

19. Fertilization by more than one sperm creates:
    a. twins.
    b. polypoid karyotype.
    c. triploid karyotype.
    d. diploid karyotype.

20. A drug prescribed for treatment of severe psoriasis, an inhibitor of cellular reproduction, and a variety of malignant neoplastic diseases is:
    a. methimazole.
    b. metaxalone.
    c. methoxy.
    d. methotrexate.

Fill-in-the-Blank

1. _____ is a nonsteroidal antiestrogen compound prescribed for the treatment of _____ cancer.

2. The most common clinical presentation of endometrial adenocarcinoma is _____.

3. An endometrium measuring greater than _____ in postmenopausal women not using hormone replacement therapy is suspect for endometrial carcinoma.

4. 3D ultrasound is used to diagnose endometrial and cervical cancers. It can detect the infiltration of cancer into the adjacent structures, _____ and _____.

5. When pelvic lesions are seen, note the presence of pelvic or abdominal _____.

6. The lower cervical lining is covered by cells that can develop into _____ carcinoma.

7. Tumors of the fallopian tube which cause profuse watery discharge are known as _____.

8. Cystic changes within the endometrium are more likely to be the result of _____, _____, or _____ but may also be seen with cancer.

9. Cervical cancer is usually asymptomatic in early stages and is often detected by _____.

10. The greatest risk factor for the development of cervical carcinoma is infection by_____.

11. Cervical cancer prognosis depends on tumor _____, tumor _____, and patient _____.

12. Along with the EV ultrasound approach, _____ and _____ methods are also used to define the cervix.

13. The appearance of a bulky cervix on ultrasound may be caused by a _____ prolapsing from the lower uterine segment.

14. Persistent trophoblastic neoplasia can occur after any pregnancy, but the greatest incidence is with _____.

15. Endovaginal sonography is essential for diagnosing persistent trophoblastic neoplasia because many of these myometrial lesions are _____.

16. Intramural fibroids undergoing degeneration may resemble invasive _____ tissue.

17. Choriocarcinoma has an absence of _____, whereas invasive mole contains it.

18. Cervical _____ results in hematometra.

19. Treatment for endometrial cancer, leiomyosarcoma, or fallopian tube carcinoma is _____.

20. Symptoms that include vaginal discharge, postcoital bleeding, bladder irritability, and low back pain are often related to _____.

Short Answer

1. Margaret, an overweight, PCOS, 64-year-old that has never married or given birth, started bleeding vaginally after being menopausal for 8 years. An EV ultrasound diagnosed a 3.3 × 2.8 × 3.1 cm heterogeneous mass in the endometrium. Provide a possible diagnosis and explain factors that lead to the diagnosis.

2. Explain GTN and its relationship to PTN.

3. Discuss the four treatment stages of cervical cancer.

IMAGE EVALUATION/PATHOLOGY

Review the images and answer the following questions.

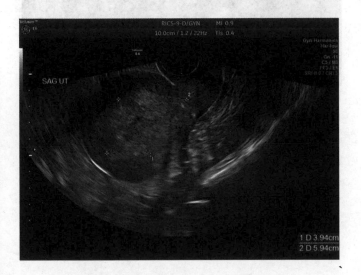

1. Identify the structure and view. What is seen between the calipers? Name the transducer used to obtain the image.

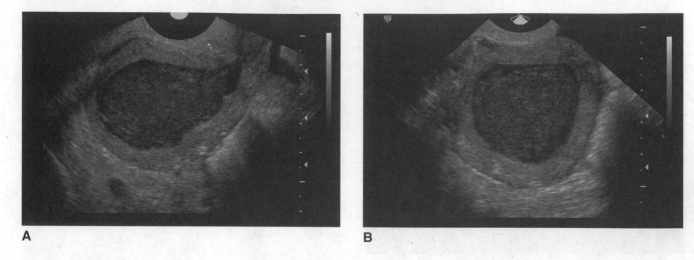

A

B

2. Describe the two images; state views and provide a diagnosis.

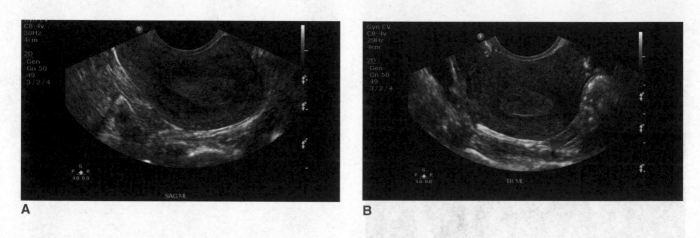

A

B

3. Explain image A and define the anatomy. Describe image B and the anatomy seen.

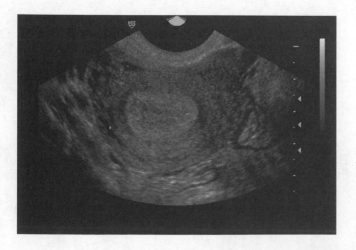

4. What is the image view? State the anatomy and pathology.

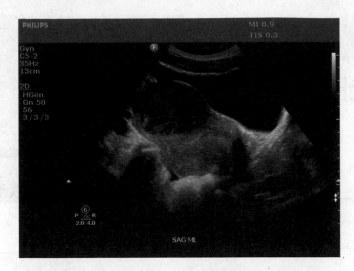

5. Define the view of image and pathology.

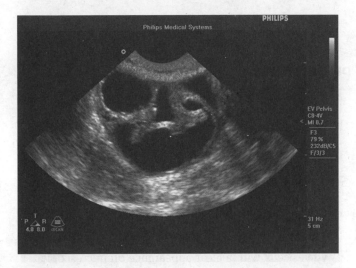

6. State the adnexal anatomy and provide a diagnosis.

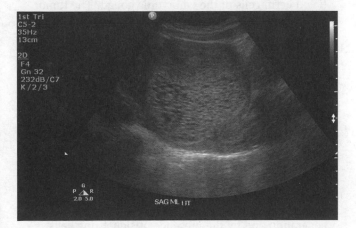

7. Describe and diagnose the anatomy within the uterine endometrium.

CHAPTER 14

Malignant Diseases of the Ovary

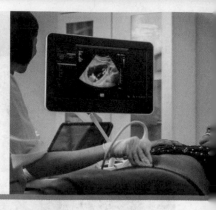

REVIEW OF GLOSSARY TERMS

Matching

Match the key terms with their definitions.

KEY TERMS

1. _____ mucinous cystadenocarcinoma

2. _____ Sertoli-Leydig cell tumors/androblastoma/ arrhenoblastoma

3. _____ Krukenberg tumor

4. _____ endometrioid tumor

5. _____ pseudomyxoma peritonei

6. _____ alpha-fetoprotein (AFP)

7. _____ clear cell adenocarcinoma

8. _____ HER2/neu

9. _____ yolk cell tumor/endodermal sinus tumor

10. _____ salpingo-oophorectomy

11. _____ lactate dehydrogenase (LDH)

12. _____ BRCA1/BRCA2

13. _____ dysgerminoma

14. _____ epithelial ovarian cancer

15. _____ serous carcinoma

16. _____ laparotomy

17. _____ struma ovarii

18. _____ Meigs syndrome

DEFINITIONS

a. Used as a tumor marker for carcinomas of embryonic origin

b. Inherited gene mutation associated with a significant increase in breast and ovarian cancer risk

c. Protein found in tumor cells, which results in an elevation of blood levels

d. Tumor marker for colon, stomach, breast, lung, some thyroid, and ovarian cancers

e. Neoplasm originating in the germ cells (ovum)

f. Neoplasm involving the surface epithelium of the female reproductive organs (ovary), which involves cells with a clear appearance on microscopic examination

g. Malignant tumor of the ovary arising from undifferentiated germ cells of the embryonic gonad. The tumor is histologically identical to seminoma found in the testicle

h. Tumor of the ovary containing epithelial or stromal elements resembling endometrial tissue. Typically arises from endometriosis and a large percentage are malignant

i. Neoplasm involving the surface epithelium of the ovary

j. Gene that produces a protein, which regulates normal cell growth found in breast and ovarian cancer cells. The identification of this protein enables determination of treatment options

k. Carcinoma of the ovary, usually metastatic from gastrointestinal cancer, marked by areas of mucoid degeneration and by the presence of signet-ring cells

l. Enzyme involved in the production of energy of the cells. Elevated levels in the blood indicates tissue damage, cancers, or other diseases

m. Surgical incision in the abdomen usually performed to evaluate the organs

19. _____ CA 125

20. _____ mucinous cystadenoma

21. _____ carcinoembryonic antigen (CEA)

22. _____ serous cystadenocarcinoma

23. _____ teratoma/teratocarcinoma

24. _____ sex cord-stromal tumors

n. The finding of pleural effusion, ascites, and an ovarian mass
o. Cystic mass filled the thick gelatinous cystic fluid
p. Large cystic ovarian mass with thick walled septations. May have internal debris layering components
q. Accumulation of mucinous material in the peritoneal cavity
r. Surgical removal of the ovary and fallopian tube
s. Type of epithelial ovarian cancer, which presents as a partially cystic mass with solid components
t. Large multilocular ovarian neoplasm with papillary projections
u. Related to the sex-cord (cord-like masses of gonadal epithelial tissue) stromal tumors seen in ovaries mostly in young adults
v. Solid ovarian mass originating from the embryonic gonadal ridges and Sertoli cells
w. Extremely rare neoplasm of the ovary containing thyroid tissue
x. A rare malignant form of a common germ cell tumor found in young adults containing fat, bone, hair, skin, and/or teeth

ANATOMY AND PHYSIOLOGY REVIEW

Image Labeling

Complete the labels in the images that follow.

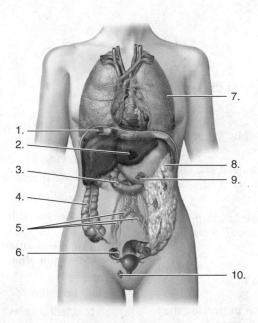

Typical metastatic sites for ovarian cancer

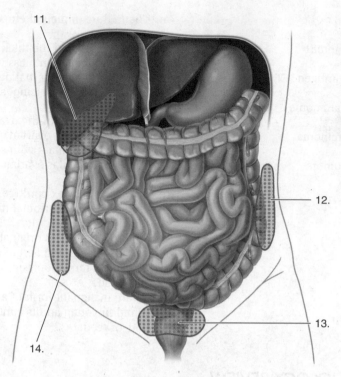

11.

12.

13.

14.

Common sites of ascites fluid collection in the peritoneum

CHAPTER REVIEW

Multiple Choice

Complete each question by circling the best answer.

1. Select the false statement.
   a. Ovarian cancer has a strong family history, making genetic screening important.
   b. Studies show that women who used oral contraceptives are at the greatest risk for developing epithelial ovarian cancer.
   c. Ovarian malignancy is a disease of low prevalence, accounting for only 5% of all female cancers.
   d. Approximately 50% of ovarian cancers occur in women in the sixth generation of life.

2. Which technique is not directed at improving the detection and outcome of ovarian cancer?
   a. Epidemiologic studies
   b. Immunologic studies
   c. Improved imaging techniques
   d. Pineal studies

3. Choose the most unlikely risk factor for developing ovarian cancer.
   a. Living in a developing country
   b. Late menopause
   c. Nulliparity
   d. Menses with early onset

4. Extended ovulatory activity, over 40 years, places women in what risk category for developing ovarian cancer?
   a. Low risk
   b. Medium risk
   c. High risk
   d. Ovulatory activity is not a factor.

5. The gene that is related to errors in the replication process resulting in overexpression:

   a. thymine

   b. HER2/neu

   c. BRCA1

   d. BRCA1

6. A characteristic of most epithelial cancers is the tendency to:

   a. display irregular borders with heterogeneous contents

   b. cause extreme, continuous pain

   c. form cystic masses with multiple septa

   d. demonstrate well-circumscribed borders

7. The major pattern of metastatic spread of ovarian malignancy is direct extension involving the neighboring organs in the pelvis, peritoneal seeding, and _____ spread.

   a. ascitic

   b. peritoneal

   c. lateral gutter

   d. lymphatic

8. Frequently, the only symptom of ovarian cancer is:

   a. right upper quadrant pain caused by ascites accumulation

   b. abdominal bloating and pain

   c. bilateral leg discomfort owing to mass encroachment of the femoral nerve

   d. urinary tract infection and vaginal bleeding

9. To increase specificity in diagnosing ovarian malignancy, laboratory values such as _____ are tested.

   a. CA 125, AFP, hCG, CEA

   b. CA 125, LDH, PET, BPT

   c. LDH, CEA, CA 51.3, APF

   d. CA 152, LDH, CD, 3D

10. What imaging method provides diagnostic value by presenting calcifications, sometimes in a curvilinear fashion, soft tissue masses, and patterns suggesting abdominal distention?

    a. Hysterography

    b. Fluoroscopy

    c. CT

    d. Plain film radiography

11. The imaging modality providing the most accurate tissue characterization regarding adnexal masses is:

    a. ultrasound, including 3D multiplanar technology

    b. CT

    c. MRI

    d. PET

12. Menopausal females utilizing HRT (hormone replacement therapy) will demonstrate:

    a. "lumpy" ovarian stroma

    b. normal-sized ovaries

    c. ovarian regression

    d. diminished ovarian blood supply

13. Ovarian malignancy screening utilizing ultrasound should consider all except:

    a. ovarian position

    b. ovarian size

    c. ovarian texture

    d. bilateral ovarian comparison

14. Metastasis to the ovary:

    a. is rare

    b. is common

    c. occurs most commonly from primary brain carcinoma

    d. causes bladder frequency

15. Compressibility of a mass while scanning can assist in differentiating bowel from malignancy and is performed by:

    a. EV ultrasound

    b. Valsalva technique

    c. "hands-on" maneuver

    d. positioning the patient in Trendelenburg

16. Nonneoplastic cystic foci of the ovary are commonly seen in _____ females and are difficult to differentiate from malignant lesions, so should be considered when determining the diagnosis.

    a. premenstrual

    b. menstruating

    c. perimenopausal

    d. menopausal

17. Epithelial ovarian cancers typically form cystic masses and:

    a. solid papillary growths

    b. reduction in ovarian volume

    c. tissue specificity used to determine benign versus malignant lesions

    d. decreased laboratory enzyme levels

18. Pseudomyxoma peritonei is defined as:

    a. illusive peritoneal ascites, which is difficult to image

    b. a type of ovarian cancer presenting as a partially cystic mass with solid components

    c. pleural effusion, ascites, and an ovarian mass

    d. the accumulation of gelatinous material in the peritoneal cavity

19. Ovarian malignancy is often associated with ascites that first accumulates in the:
    a. right upper quadrant
    b. bilateral paracolic gutters
    c. dependent portion of the peritoneal cavity
    d. splenic flexure

20. Color Doppler of malignant lesions frequently demonstrates:
    a. reduced vascular patterns
    b. prominent flow in the septations
    c. peripheral vascular patterns
    d. no vascular patterns

Fill-in-the-Blank

1. Ovarian masses, whether malignant or benign, can result in _____ of the ovary.

2. A large number of patients with ovarian malignancy present with or develop _____ bleeding.

3. Two inherited gene mutations related to an increase of breast and ovarian cancer are _____ and _____.

4. A Krukenberg tumor is a cancerous tumor of the _____ and usually metastasizes from _____ cancer.

5. The effect of ovulation is known to cause increased inflammation and wound healing owing to repeated trauma to the ovarian _____.

6. Ascites associated with ovarian malignancy collects in the _____ and _____, mostly on the _____ side.

7. Ovarian cancer is mostly a disease of _____ menopausal and _____ menopausal women.

8. Ovarian cancer is the most common tumor responsible for _____ malignancy in women.

9. Symptoms of abnormal _____ activity are sometimes a clue to the presence of an ovarian malignancy that is hormonally active.

10. Benign processes, such as _____, _____, and even pancreatitis result in an increased CA 125, as does ovarian cancer.

11. AFP is alpha-fetoprotein; LDH is _____; CEA is _____; and hCG is _____.

12. A CT examination can demonstrate pelvic sidewall masses, lymph node enlargement in the retroperitoneum, liver metastases, and calcifications, especially when _____ and _____ contrast is given.

13. Although it cannot always distinguish a malignant process from benign, _____ remains the diagnostic method of choice as a screening technique for adnexal processes.

14. The effective method to investigate for ovarian cancer includes _____ ultrasound, _____ examination, and the tumor marker, _____.

15. To determine pelvic mass from possible bowel, _____ must be identified.

16. PET should only be used in a select group of patients in whom both _____ and _____ have failed to yield unequivocal results.

17. Fallopian tube neoplasms are rare and malignant. These lesions are mistaken for _____ malignancies.

18. Ovarian cancer is one of the most lethal forms of cancer owing to _____.

19. Exploratory _____ remains the gold standard in the visualization of adnexal malignancy.
_____ imaging is most helpful in staging ovarian cancer.

20. Eighty percent of ovarian malignancies originate from the _____ covering the ovaries.

Short Answer

1. Discuss factors that determine the prognosis of ovarian cancer.

2. In what way is breast cancer related to ovarian cancer?

3. Discuss laboratory assays utilized in the detection of ovarian cancer. Consider increased levels as well as declines.

4. A 62-year-old menopausal woman complains to her gynecologist of dull pain in her inferior pelvis. State current diagnostic tools available to investigate and determine her condition.

IMAGE EVALUATION/PATHOLOGY

Review the images and answer the following questions.

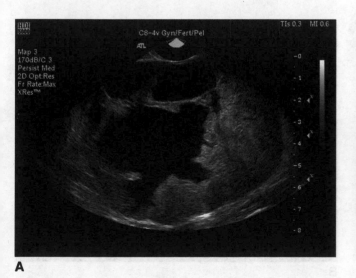

A

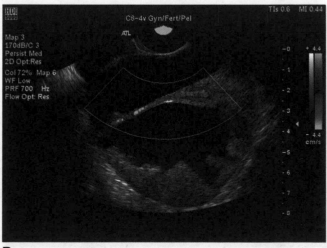

B

1. Name the structure visualized in images A and B. What transducer was used to obtain these images?

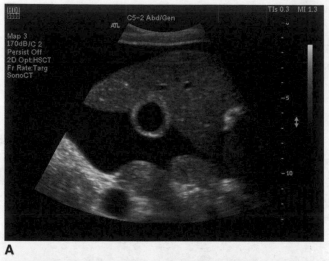

A

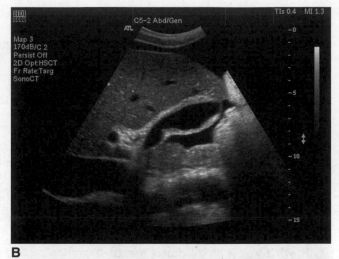

B

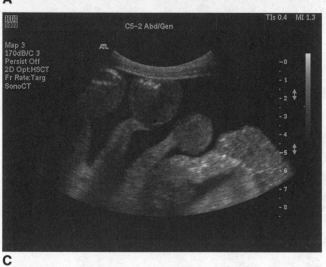

C

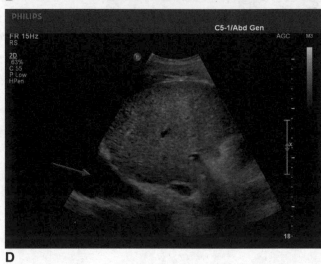

D

2. Explain the pathology in images A through D.

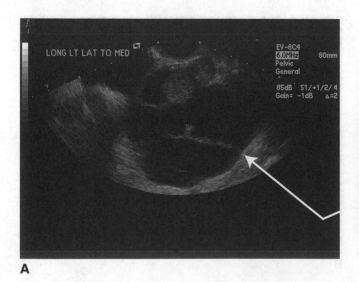

A

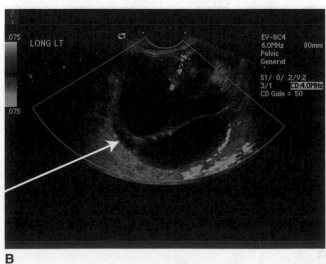

B

3. Describe the two images. Offer a diagnosis.

CHAPTER 15

Pelvic Inflammatory Disease and Endometriosis

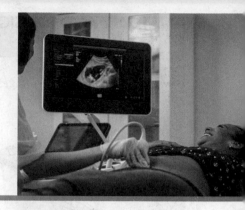

REVIEW OF GLOSSARY TERMS

Matching

Match the key terms with their definitions.

KEY TERMS

1. _____ pyosalpinx

2. _____ oophoritis

3. _____ tubo-ovarian abscess (TOA)

4. _____ tubo-ovarian complex

5. _____ adenomyosis

6. _____ Fitz-Hugh-Curtis syndrome

7. _____ dysmenorrhea

8. _____ salpingitis

9. _____ endometriosis

10. _____ myometritis

11. _____ pelvic inflammatory disease (PID)

12. _____ endometritis

13. _____ endometrioma

14. _____ parametritis

15. _____ peritonitis

16. _____ dyspareunia

DEFINITIONS

a. Presence of endometrial glands and tissue found in the uterine wall
b. Painful menstruation
c. Painful intercourse
d. Implants of endometrial tissue outside the uterus
e. Blood-filled cyst located on the ovary, which is the result of endometriosis
f. Bacterial infection of the endometrium with potential extension into the surrounding (parametrial) tissues
g. Rare complication of PID resulting in the development of liver adhesions owing to the inflammatory exudates
h. Myometrial inflammation
i. Infection of the ovaries
j. Infection of the connective tissue surrounding the uterus
k. Infection of the female reproductive tract
l. Pus within the fallopian tube
m. Infection of the fallopian tube
n. Infection found in the late stages of PID resulting in the inability to differentiate tubal and ovarian structures
o. Ability to identify the ovary and tube in the presence of adhesions or infection
p. Infection of the peritoneum

ANATOMY AND PHYSIOLOGY REVIEW

Image Labeling

Complete the labels in the images that follow.

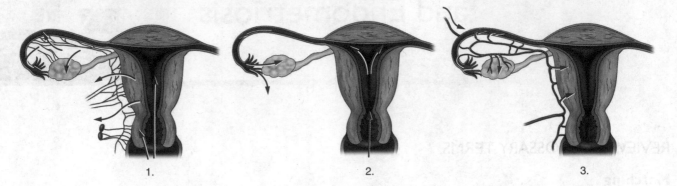

Microorganisms and pathways of pelvic infections

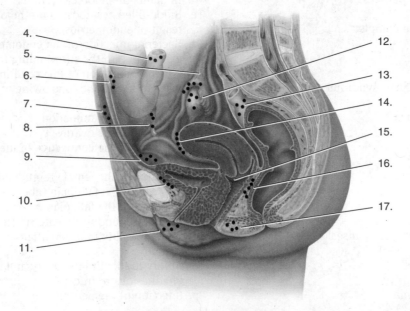

Common sites of endometriosis

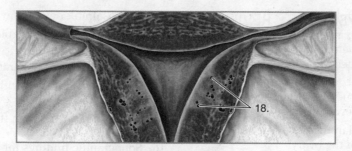

Process involving endometrial cell growth into the myometrium

CHAPTER REVIEW

Multiple Choice

Complete each question by circling the best answer.

1. Pelvic inflammatory disease is:
   a. scarring of the fallopian tube epithelium owing to injury
   b. thickening and redistribution of the endometrium owing to injury or infection
   c. a process of heavy, painful bleeding caused by inflammation
   d. infection of the female genital tract causing diffuse inflammation

2. One incident of PID can increase the risk of tubal factor infertility and ectopic pregnancy:
   a. two times
   b. four times
   c. six times
   d. 10 times

3. Bacterial vaginosis (BV) is the most common infection of the ____ in reproductive-age women.
   a. lower genital tract
   b. upper genital tract
   c. fallopian tubes
   d. uterine endometrium

4. Early sonographic findings of pelvic inflammatory disease are:
   a. concentrated complex adnexa
   b. acute inflammatory process
   c. purulent edema
   d. often nonspecific

5. A normal fallopian tube:
   a. demonstrates endosalpingeal folds
   b. is not visualized with ultrasound
   c. is an elongated oval structure
   d. is hypoechoic.

6. Fitz-Hugh-Curtis syndrome is caused by peritonitis and includes what organ:
   a. Pancreas
   b. Spleen
   c. Liver
   d. Ovaries

7. Acute PID sonographic findings are all except:
   a. edematous fallopian tube wall, large amount of pelvic free fluid
   b. enlarged ovaries
   c. purulent exudate escaping the tube
   d. sharp uterine borders

8. When seen in cross-section, a hydrosalpinx may exhibit as:
   a. an echoic adnexal structure
   b. the "beads on a string" sign
   c. a "chocolate cyst"
   d. "ground glass"

9. Define tubo-ovarian complex:

    a. Tubo-ovarian complex refers to the affected ovary and tube that are adherent to one another, but their individual architecture is still identifiable on ultrasound.

    b. Ovarian and tubal structures cannot be seen separately on ultrasound evaluation.

    c. Pus within the fallopian tube and infection of the peritoneal covering of the ovary

    d. Infection of the female reproductive tract

10. Chronic progression of endometriosis can lead to all but the following:

    a. Severe cyclic pelvic pain

    b. Infertility

    c. Simple cysts

    d. Endometrial invasion of organs

11. Endometriosis is known to affect:

    a. all menstruating females

    b. reproductive-age females

    c. perimenopausal females

    d. postmenopausal females

12. Endometriosis ____ transforms into malignancy.

    a. rarely

    b. never

    c. usually

    d. always

13. Introduction of an IUD may elevate the risk for PID following insertion for:

    a. 1 to 3 days

    b. up to 3 weeks

    c. 5 to 10 days

    d. 1 month

14. Endometriomas appear sonographically thick-walled, spherical masses, and frequently (95% of the time) displaying:

    a. low-level internal echoes ("ground glass" appearance)

    b. a singular simple cystic appearance

    c. hypoechoic "bubble" appearance

    d. internal finger-like projections

15. Hydrosalpinx develops when:

    a. ovaries enlarge and blockage of the fallopian tube occurs distally

    b. pelvic infection migrates through the uterus

    c. fluid accumulates within a scarred, obstructed fallopian tube

    d. pus develops within the infected fallopian tube

16. Sonographic findings for adenomyosis are all except:

    a. an asymmetrically enlarged uterus

    b. heterogeneous myometrial echotexture

    c. peripheral uterine calcific deposits

    d. myometrial cysts

17. Endometriomas image as:

    a. a complex mass with color flow signal

    b. smooth-walled structures with low-level internal echoes

    c. anechoic

    d. a tubular purulent structure

18. Choose the correct statement regarding pelvic inflammatory disease.

    a. Early stages demonstrate a variable appearance and an enlarged uterus with indistinct margins.

    b. Salpingitis displaying thin-walled tubes with pyosalpinx

    c. Normal ovarian dimensions with ill-defined tissue planes

    d. No pelvic free fluid will be seen.

19. The most effective treatment for patients suffering from severe endometriosis who do not respond to conservative surgical management and medical therapies is:

    a. narcotic analgesics

    b. aromatase inhibitors, selective progesterone receptor modulators, and tumor necrosis factor-alpha inhibitors

    c. angiogenic ablation

    d. oophorectomy and hormonal medical management

20. Endometriosis can implant in all areas except the:

    a. ovary

    b. groin

    c. posterior cul-de-sac

    d. pelvic lymph nodes

Fill-in-the-Blank

1. The most likely area for PID to develop is _____, also known as _____.

2. The three major sequelae of PID are _____, _____, and _____.

3. A fallopian tube affected with PID demonstrates a _____ sign when imaged in cross-section.

4. Clinical findings that include right-sided pleuritic pain and right-sided upper quadrant pain and tenderness on palpitation related to PID is called _____.

5. PID of the uterine myometrial endometrial junction appears _____, and the endometrium may be thickened and heterogeneous and contain _____ within the cavity.

6. Escape of purulent exudate beyond the fallopian tube results in _____ complex.

7. The presence of endometrial glands and tissues in the uterine wall is _____.

8. Endometriosis nodules may vary from _____ echoic to _____ echoic in appearance and may be either _____ in the case of recent hemorrhage or _____ secondary to fibrosis.

9. Focal ovarian endometriosis appears on ultrasound examination as cystic structures called _____.

10. Endometriosis can be diffuse or _____.

11. The sonographic appearance of adenomyosis lacks a discrete _____ within the myometrium.

12. Adenomyosis is generally treated _____.

13. _____ may be difficult to differentiate from an ovarian cyst or small cystadenoma.

14. _____ is infection of the ovary(ies).

15. A round mass-like calcific structure with edge shadowing and peripheral vascularization is a _____.

16. An endometrioma associated with the urinary bladder causes _____ symptoms.

17. A highly sensitive and specific imaging method for diagnosing adenomyosis is _____.

18. An elevated white blood count, vaginal secretions, elevated erythrocyte sedimentation rate, and C-reactive protein is an indication of _____.

19. If color Doppler flow is visualized within an endometrioma, _____ must be suspected.

20. Adenomyosis usually affects the _____ portion of the uterus.

Short Answer

1. Discuss the migration and stages of PID.

2. A 19-year-old presents to her gynecologist with an off-white discharge and 1 week of low pelvic pain following spring break from college. She admits to being sexually active. What additional symptoms would be helpful to diagnose PID?

3. A strong family history of endometriosis existed in a 28-year-old with constant dull pelvic pain that worsened during menstruation. Explain endometriosis, symptoms, and its stages.

4. A G3 P3 40-year-old married female, who is faithful to her husband, presents with complaints of continual tenderness in the pelvis and erratic bleeding. Her physician reports guarding and uterine enlargement upon physical examination. Based on symptoms and examination observation, is PID, endometriosis, or adenomyosis a more accurate pre-imaging diagnosis?

IMAGE EVALUATION/PATHOLOGY

Review the images and answer the following questions.

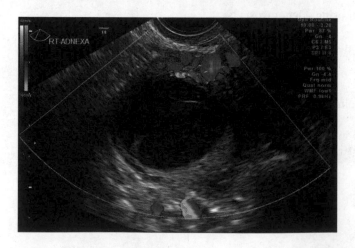

1. Diagnose the image.

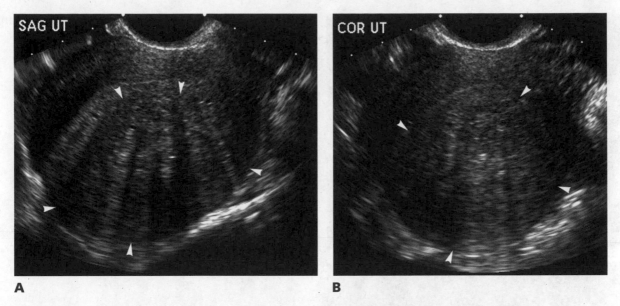

2. What do the coronal and sagittal views of the uterus demonstrate?

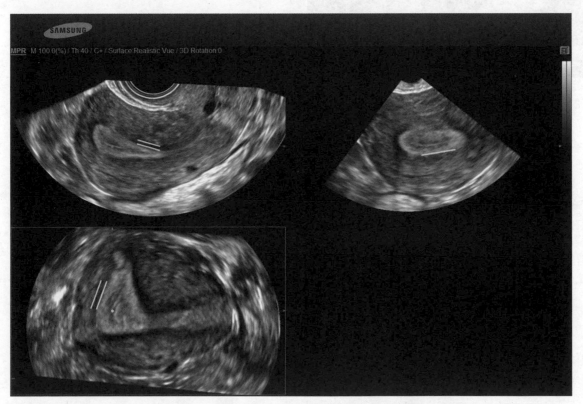

3. Name the type of imaging. Are the junctional zone images normal or irregular?

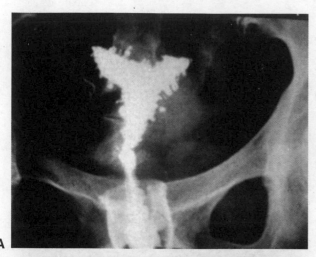

A

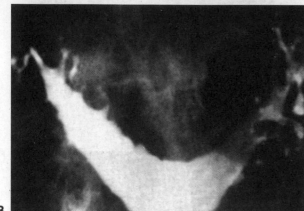

B

4. Name the type of imaging. Diagnose the study and explain the findings.

CHAPTER 16

Imaging the Intrauterine Device

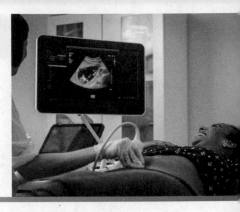

REVIEW OF GLOSSARY TERMS

Matching

Match the key terms with their definitions.

KEY TERMS

1. _____ ovicidal

2. _____ displacement

3. _____ cornu

4. _____ chorioamnionitis

5. _____ intrauterine contraceptive device (IUD or IUCD)

6. _____ fragmentation

7. _____ embedment

8. _____ intracavitary

9. _____ levonorgestrel (LNG-IUD)

10. _____ perforation

11. _____ expulsion

12. _____ incrustation

13. _____ transcervical tubal occlusion device

14. _____ radiopaque

DEFINITIONS

a. Within an organ or body cavity

b. Product inserted into the uterine cavity as a mechanism to prevent pregnancy or deliver hormones

c. IUCD with synthetic progesterone embedded in a reservoir surrounding the shaft

d. Relating to or causing death of an ovum

e. Material or tissue that blocks the passage of X-rays, with a bone or near-bone density. A radiopaque structure is white or nearly white on conventional X-rays.

f. Horn-shaped anatomical structure (as of the uterus). The uterine cornua are where the uterus and fallopian tubes meet.

g. Penetration into the myometrium, but not through the serosa

h. Penetration through the myometrium and serosa, either partially or completely with migration into the intraperitoneal cavity

i. Located either partially or completely through the external cervical os

j. IUCD that is rotated from the normal transverse position or located away from the fundus and within the lower uterine segment or cervix or lacks deployment of the wings

k. Form of permanent contraception using metallic coils or a silicone plug to obstruct the fallopian tubes

l. Formation of calcium carbonate deposits on or near the IUD, demonstrated as uneven echoes surrounding the normal IUD echoes

m. IUD that has been broken during expulsion or removal, including embedded removal strings

n. Serious condition in pregnant women in which the membranes that surround the fetus and the amniotic fluid are infected by bacteria

ANATOMY AND PHYSIOLOGY REVIEW

Image Labeling

Complete the labels in the images that follow.

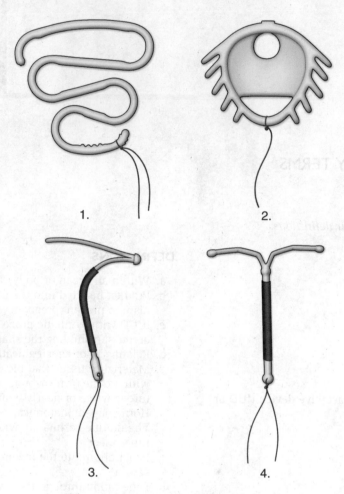

1.

2.

3.

4.

U.S. intrauterine devices

CHAPTER REVIEW

Multiple Choice

Complete each question by circling the best answer.

1. Select the IUCD that has never been marketed in the United States.
   a. Copper IUCD
   b. Lippes loop
   c. Chinese ring
   d. Levonorgestrel IUCD

2. Choose the false statement.
   a. IUCD arms measure between 20 and 30 mm.
   b. Polyethylene monofilament retrieval strings attach to the base of the IUCD stem.
   c. An IUCD consists of a T-shaped polyethylene frame.
   d. An IUCD shaft length measures 30 to 36 mm.

3. A mispositioned or expelled IUCD can be owing to:
   a. type of IUCD
   b. gravida status of the female
   c. age of the female
   d. congenital malformation

4. Expulsion risk of an IUCD is greatest in the:
   a. first month following insertion
   b. first week following insertion
   c. first year of use
   d. first 6 months of use

5. Displacement of the IUCD occurs when an IUCD:
   a. has been broken during expulsion or removal
   b. is rotated from the normal transverse position
   c. is completely through the external cervical os
   d. causes the death of an ovum

6. IUCD position is best documented by:
   a. CT
   b. 3D and 4D sonography
   c. X-ray
   d. 2D sonography

7. The optimal position of the copper or hormone-releasing IUCD is:
   a. in the fundal portion of the endometrial cavity with the wings extending to the uterine cornua
   b. within the uterus 2 cm from the uterine fundus to the superior endometrial cavity
   c. within the uterus 2 cm from the internal cervical os
   d. in the fundal portion with the wings deployed in a "T" or "Y" position

8. If the IUCD is visible or can be felt that the external cervical os, it is labeled as:
   a. perforated
   b. embedded
   c. displaced
   d. partially expulsed

9. IUCD perforation occurs more frequently in:
   a. gravida 0 females
   b. a fibroid uterus
   c. gravida 4 to 8 females
   d. lactating patients or those who have given birth within the past 6 months

10. Select the incorrect statement.
    a. Embedment of an IUCD often occurs at the time of insertion.
    b. The copper IUCD releases levonorgestrel ions.
    c. Embedment of an IUCD occurs through gradual penetration in the uterine wall.
    d. Patients with a displaced IUCD may be asymptomatic but present with a missing IUCD string.

11. Silicone impregnated matrix devices used for permanent birth control appear on sonography as:
    a. dual coils
    b. bulbous
    c. a 2-cm linear echogenic focus near the uterine cornu
    d. echogenic foci located on the lateral borders of the uterine cornua

12. Uterine perforation by an IUCD may cause all except:
    a. vaginal bleeding
    b. no symptoms
    c. tubal occlusion
    d. abdominal pain

13. Essure© is a permanent birth control that is no longer used in the United States. When used, where was it inserted?
    a. Fallopian tube
    b. Ovarian artery
    c. Cervix
    d. Fornix

14. The risk of a pregnancy in a female with an IUCD is:
    a. fetal perforation
    b. endometrial perforation
    c. multiple pregnancies
    d. ectopic pregnancy

Fill-in-the-Blank

1. The two IUCD types marketed in the United States, which provide reversible contraception are _____ and _____.

2. An IUCD that moves from the uterine endometrium though the cervical os is known as an IUCD _____.

3. Transcervical tubal devices are a form of contraception introduced for women to achieve _____ contraception.

4. The IUCD string is also known as _____ string.

5. Leaving an IUCD in place with a viable pregnancy increases the rates of spontaneous _____, bleeding, premature _____ , preterm delivery, _____, and fetal congenital malformations.

6. The wings of the displaced IUCD often become _____ or can even _____ the uterine wall.

7. All types of IUCDs should be located in the _____ portion of the endometrial cavity.

8. A properly positioned IUCD should appear as a _____ echogenic structure in the endometrium.

9. The older copper IUCDs can decrease in effectiveness owing to _____ (calcification).

10. A spiral shaped IUCD is a _____.

Short Answer

1. A patient who had an IUD placed 2 years ago is now unable to locate the string during her monthly string check. What may cause the inability to detect the string, and what is the best method to reveal the IUD position?

2. A female complaining of severe abdomen pain presents to the emergency department. Laboratory tests and routine abdomen/pelvis radiographs are ordered to assist with diagnosis. The inferior mid-pelvis radiograph demonstrates a "bright" circular artifact in the inferior mid-pelvis. Provide a likely explanation for the artifact.

IMAGE EVALUATION/PATHOLOGY

Review the images and answer the following questions.

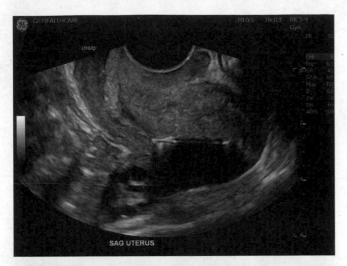

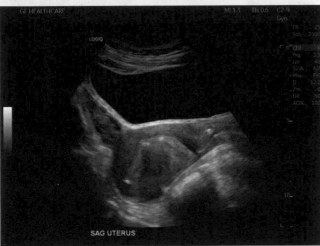

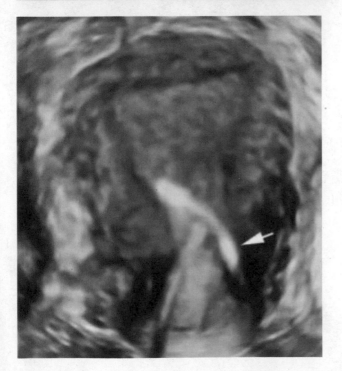

1. Explain the anatomy in the image. What is the view? What imaging method was used to collect this image?

2. Explain the anatomy in the image. What is the view? What imaging method was used to collect this image?

3. Analyze the image of the lower uterine segment and cervix. Explain.

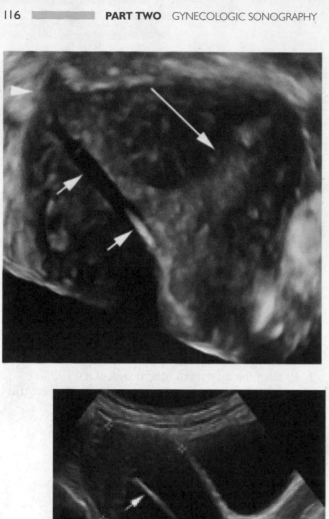

4. Identify the anatomy and describe the IUCD position.

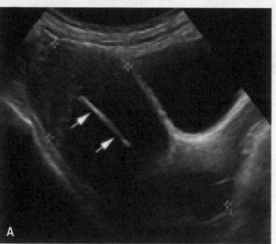

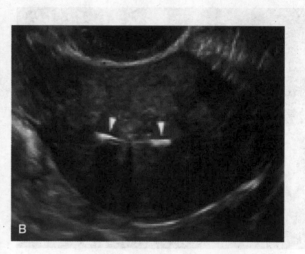

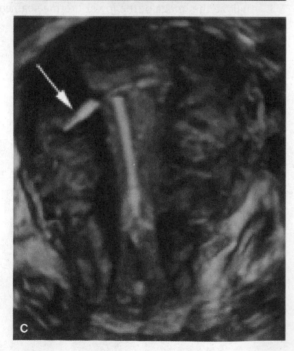

5. Diagnose the three images.

PART THREE

OBSTETRIC SONOGRAPHY

CHAPTER 17

The Use of Ultrasound in the First Trimester

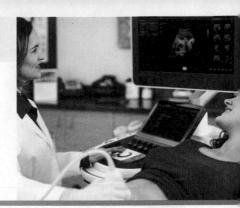

REVIEW OF GLOSSARY TERMS

Matching

Match the key terms with their definitions.

KEY TERMS

1. _____ estrogen

2. _____ mean sac diameter (MSD)

3. _____ Naegele rule

4. _____ decidualization

5. _____ luteinizing hormone

6. _____ umbilical vesicle (synonym: yolk sac)

7. _____ estimated date of delivery (EDD)

8. _____ LMP

9. _____ spermatozoon (plural: spermatozoa)

10. _____ crown–rump length (CRL)

11. _____ human chorionic gonadotropin (hCG)

12. _____ progesterone

13. _____ corpus luteum

14. _____ gravidity

15. _____ parity

16. _____ conceptus

17. _____ gestational sac

DEFINITIONS

a. Minimizing the risk of ultrasound-induced bioeffects by controlling acoustic output, scan modes, machine settings, and duration of exposure

b. Membrane enclosing the amniotic cavity and embryo or fetus

c. Abnormal number of chromosomes

d. Early gestation consisting of a thin outer layer of cells (trophoblast), a fluid-filled cavity, and an inner cell mass (embryoblast)

e. Membrane around the chorionic cavity, made up of trophoblast cells and extraembryonic mesoderm

f. Bud-like outward growths from the trophoblast, some of which will give rise to the fetal portion of the placenta

g. Duration of pregnancy counted from fertilization (conception) expressed in hours or days. Also called embryonic age or postovulatory age

h. Product of fertilization including all stages from zygote to fetus

i. Progesterone-secreting structure formed by a follicle after releasing its oocyte

j. Measurement of longest axis of an embryo; determines gestational age

k. Due date, calculated by adding 280 days to the first day of the last menstrual period. Also called estimated date of confinement (EDC)

l. Changes in the endometrium to allow implantation of a blastocyst

m. Group of hormones, primarily produced in the ovaries, which affect secondary sex characteristics and the menstrual cycle

n. Penetration of an oocyte by a sperm to form a diploid zygote

o. Hormone produced in the anterior pituitary, which stimulates the maturation of ovarian follicles

18. _____ morula

19. _____ conceptual age

20. _____ gestational age (GA, synonym: menstrual age)

21. _____ pregnancy-associated plasma protein A (PAPP-A)

22. _____ chorionic villi

23. _____ amnion

24. _____ gamete

25. _____ oocyte

26. _____ chorion

27. _____ follicle-stimulating hormone (FSH)

28. _____ nuchal translucency (NT)

29. _____ blastocyst

30. _____ second trimester

31. _____ fertilization

32. _____ third trimester

33. _____ zygote

34. _____ ALARA (as low as reasonably achievable) principle

35. _____ first trimester

p. Haploid cell that when merged with a gamete from the opposite sex creates a diploid zygote

q. Duration of pregnancy counted from the first day of the last menstrual period, expressed in weeks and days or fractions of weeks. A pregnancy typically lasts about 280 days or 40 weeks, counted from the first day of the last menstrual period and is commonly divided into three trimesters.

r. First sonographic evidence of an intrauterine pregnancy, the fluid-filled blastocyst

s. Number of times a woman has been pregnant

t. Hormone produced by trophoblast cells of the blastocyst, which extends the life of the corpus luteum in the ovary. Most pregnancy tests are based on the detection of hCG.

u. First day of last menstrual period

v. A hormone produced in the anterior pituitary, which triggers ovulation in females

w. Average mean diameter of the gestational sac used to determine GA

x. Solid cluster of undifferentiated cells formed by repeated cleavage of the single cell that resulted from the fusion of two gametes

y. Subcutaneous fluid in the posterior region of the neck of embryos and fetuses up to 14 weeks GA. Abnormally large nuchal translucencies have been associated with a higher risk of chromosomal and structural abnormalities.

z. Female gamete, aka ovum or egg

aa. Protein produced by the trophoblasts. Abnormal levels of PAPP-A may be associated with an increased risk of chromosomal abnormalities.

bb. Hormone produced by the corpus luteum and the placenta

cc. Third trimester—28 weeks to delivery

dd. Structure within the cavity of the blastocyst, which provides nourishment to the embryo and produces its first blood cells. The secondary umbilical vesicle (yolk sac) is the first structure to be sonographically identified within the gestational sac.

ee. Calculation to find a patient's EDD:
(1) Take LMP
(2) Add 1 year
(3) Subtract 3 months
(4) Add 7 days

ff. Single cell resulting from the fusion of two gametes

gg. Summary of a woman's pregnancy outcomes. The most common description of parity is expressed in four numbers. The first is the number of term deliveries; the second number is the number of preterm deliveries (usually after 24 weeks GA); the third is the number of other pregnancies and includes both spontaneous and therapeutic abortions; the fourth number is the woman's living children.

hh. First trimester—0 day (first day of last menstrual period) to end of the 13th week

ii. Second trimester—14 weeks to the end of the 27th week

ANATOMY AND PHYSIOLOGY REVIEW

Image Labeling

Complete the labels in the images that follow.

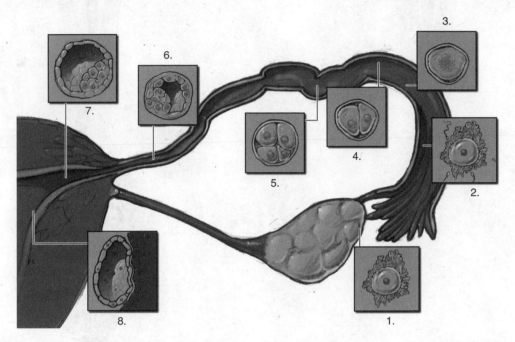

Fertilization and cell division—*Label each box insert and state hours or days of development.*

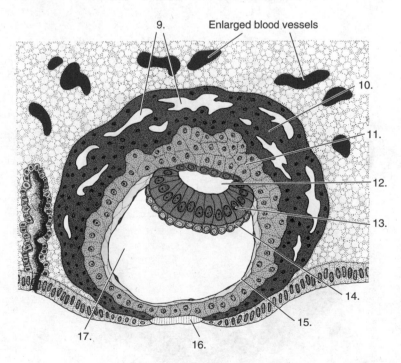

Nine-day human blastocyst—*Label*

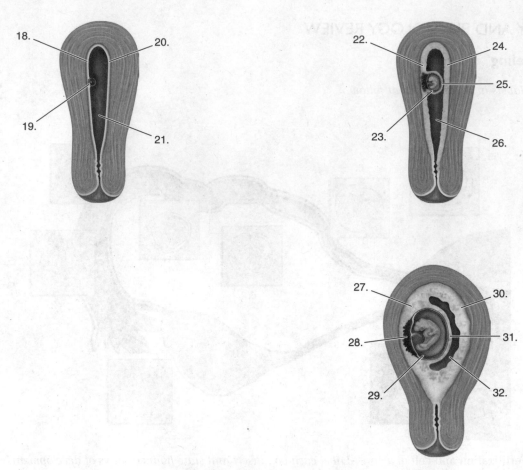

Uterine embryo implantation—*Label*

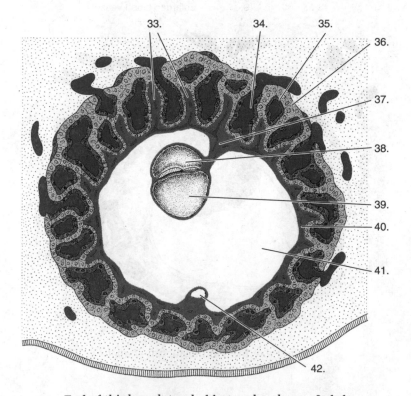

End of third week trophoblast and embryo—*Label*

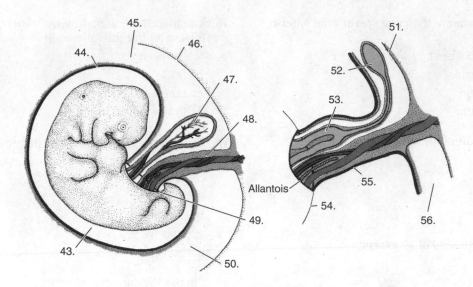

Five-week embryo—*Label*

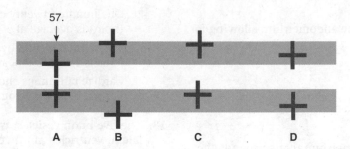

NT measurement—*Select the letter depicting correct measurement method.*

CHAPTER REVIEW

Multiple Choice

Complete each question by circling the best answer.

1. A normal gestation lasts approximately:
   a. 200 days
   b. 280 days
   c. 9 months
   d. 9.5 months

2. Ultrasound in the first trimester is mostly performed to demonstrate:
   a. GA
   b. EDD and FSH
   c. EDD, GA, and likelihood of continuing to term
   d. to evaluate a corpus luteum and EDD

3. The head of the sperm cells contains _____, which house enzymes allowing for penetration of the outer layer of the ovum.
   a. mitochondria
   b. nucleus
   c. acrosome
   d. seminiferous fluid

4. The _____ hormone triggers ovulation.
   a. luteinizing
   b. hCG
   c. follicle-stimulating
   d. estrogen

5. What does not assist the ova to move into and through the fallopian tube?
   a. Fimbriae
   b. Contractile walls
   c. Cilia
   d. Infundibulum

6. Fertilization generally occurs in the _____ portion of the fallopian tube.
   a. ampullary
   b. isthmic
   c. fimbriated
   d. interstitial

7. What prevents more than one sperm from entering an ovum?
   a. Cytotrophoblast shell
   b. Zona pellucida
   c. Exocoelomic
   d. Mitochondria

8. A cluster or ball of forming cells is a:
   a. zygote
   b. conceptus
   c. morula
   d. trophoblast

9. A blastocyst consists of all except:
   a. blastocele
   b. trophoblast
   c. embryoblast
   d. blastocyte

10. Preparatory change in the endometrium allowing for implantation is:
    a. decidualization
    b. basal reaction
    c. implantation window
    d. trophoblastic

11. The portion of the endometrium that surrounds the blastocyst is:
    a. decidua parietalis
    b. decidua capsularis
    c. decidua basalis
    d. decidua vera

12. The yolk sac becomes part of the embryonic gut and contributes to:
    a. digestive, respiratory, and urogenital development
    b. primitive colon and neurologic development
    c. genital and cardiac development
    d. amnion and fluid development

13. The first structure seen sonographically within the uterus in early pregnancy is the:
    a. yolk sac
    b. blastocyst
    c. amniotic cavity
    d. chorionic sac

14. At what age have the rudimentary forms of all embryonic organs and structures developed?
    a. 8 weeks GA
    b. Almost 11 weeks menstrual/GA
    c. 10 weeks postconception
    d. 5 weeks from the LMP

15. The placenta will mature from early pregnancy to release all but the following:
    a. Estrogen
    b. hCG
    c. Luteinizing hormone
    d. Progesterone

16. Sonography may detect a blastocyst embedded in the decidua as early as _____ after conception.
    a. 11 days
    b. 21 days
    c. 2 weeks + 4 days
    d. 2 weeks

17. Choose the correct statement.
    a. The primitive heart begins to beat about 27 days after conception.
    b. One hundred twenty cardiac beats per minute (bpm) is average at 5 weeks of age.
    c. The normal resting heart rate of a third-trimester fetus is 110 to 160 beats per minute (bpm).
    d. Cardiac pulsations should be documented in all normal embryos 8 mm or larger.

18. The five brain vesicles, which will become the lateral ventricles, third ventricle, and the upper and lower parts of the fourth ventricle, and the connections between them develop from the:
    a. prosencephalon and rhombencephalon
    b. telencephalon
    c. diencephalon
    d. mesencephalon and midbrain

19. The most accurate measurement for dating in early pregnancy is the:
    a. mean sac diameter
    b. maximal sac diameter
    c. LMP
    d. CRL

20. When the NT measurement is combined with _____, the detection rate for trisomy 21 increases to 86%.
    a. EDC
    b. PAPP-A and free beta-hCG
    c. biochemical markers
    d. human chorionic gonadotropin

Fill-in-the-Blank

1. Spontaneous pregnancy loss most often happens in the _____.

2. Gametes are _____ cells with _____ chromosomes.

3. The whip-like tails of sperm contain _____.

4. The pituitary gland produces _____.

5. A ruptured follicle, or corpus luteum, releases _____.

6. Once the ovum is fertilized, the structure is called a single diploid cell, _____, or _____.

7. _____ hours after fertilization, rapid cell division occurs. It is known as _____.

8. The developing cluster of cells travels through the fallopian tube and reaches the uterus about _____ days after fertilization.

9. The two endometrial layers are a thin _____ layer adjacent to the myometrium and a functional layer of _____.

10. The implantation window begins _____ days after ovulation and lasts approximately _____ days.

11. Nourishment from the endometrial glands cross the _____ and enter the _____.

12. A blastocyst's inner cell mass differentiates into two layers: thick _____ adjacent to the trophoblast and thin _____ facing the blastocele.

13. The first visualized structure within the gestational sac is the _____.

14. First blood cells to the embryo are produced by the _____ and are transferred to and fro through the _____ veins and arteries.

15. The embryonic disc contains _____ germ cell layers from which all future organs and _____ are derived.

16. Fetal stage begins following the _____ period after about _____.

17. Fetal placenta occupies the _____ portion of the endometrium, leaving the basal layer intact.

18. The double sac sign is developed by two layers of decidua, _____ and _____.

19. A 5-week yolk sac measures about _____ mm in diameter and enlarges to _____ mm at 11 weeks, then disappears by _____ weeks GA.

20. The primitive fetal heart begins beating about _____ after conception.

Short Answer

1. Explain the role of the uterine endometrium at implantation.

2. Discuss and describe quantitative and qualitative pregnancy test results.

3. Explain early sonographic intrauterine pregnancy findings and correlate them with dates.

4. Define the necessary components of a first-trimester sonogram based on the AIUM *Practice Guideline for the Performance of Obstetric Ultrasound Examinations*.

IMAGE EVALUATION/PATHOLOGY

Review the images and answer the following questions.

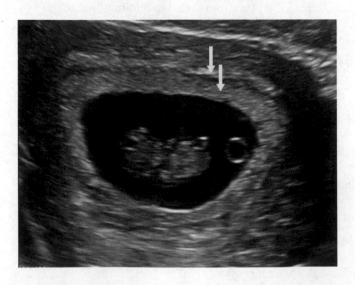

1. Name the anatomy the two arrows point at.

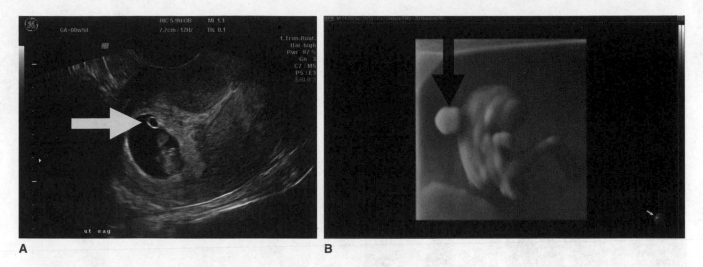

A

B

2. Name the anatomy that the arrows are directed toward. Explain the image acquisition method for the left and the right image.

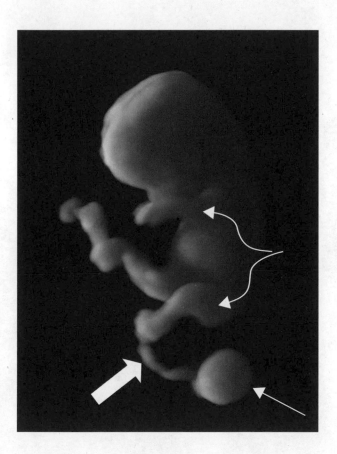

3. What do the thick, thin, and curved arrows point toward?

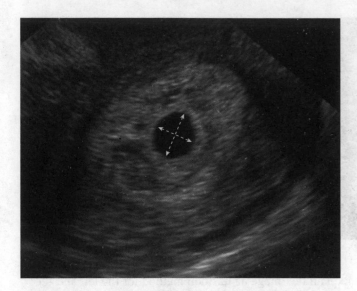

4. Explain the image.

CHAPTER 18

Sonographic Evaluation of First-Trimester Complications

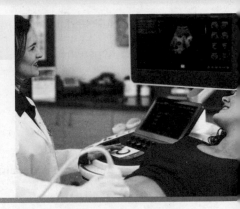

REVIEW OF GLOSSARY TERMS

Matching

Match the key terms with their definitions.

KEY TERMS

1. _____ anemia

2. _____ inevitable abortion

3. _____ complete hydatidiform mole

4. _____ toxemia of pregnancy

5. _____ abortion

6. _____ gestational trophoblastic neoplasia

7. _____ tachycardia

8. _____ anembryonic pregnancy

9. _____ hyperthyroidism

10. _____ triploid, triploidy

11. _____ chorionic villus sampling

12. _____ missed abortion

13. _____ partial hydatidiform mole

14. _____ gestational trophoblastic disease

15. _____ respiratory insufficiency

16. _____ amniocentesis

17. _____ hydatidiform mole

18. _____ threatened abortion, threatened miscarriage

DEFINITIONS

a. Spontaneous or induced termination of an early pregnancy and expulsion of fetal and placental tissues

b. Invasive procedure in which a quantity of amniotic fluid is removed from the amniotic sac for analysis of the fetal cells or for the presence of certain chemicals in the fluid itself. Amniocentesis may also be performed as a palliative measure in patients with severe polyhydramnios.

c. Pregnancy that has failed prior to the development of an identifiable embryo, or in which embryonic tissue has been resorbed after early embryo demise

d. Deficiency of red blood cells

e. Empty gestational sac seen in an anembryonic pregnancy

f. Abnormally slow heart rate

g. Invasive procedure in which the chorionic villi of an early pregnancy are removed for analysis

h. Abnormal fertilization of an oocyte that contains no maternal chromosomes, resulting in the proliferation of swollen chorionic villi and the absence of identifiable embryonic structures

i. Spectrum of disorders that begin at fertilization and involve abnormal proliferation of the trophoblasts that in a normal pregnancy would have gone on to form the placenta. Gestational trophoblastic disease may become invasive and become malignant and metastasize.

j. Invasive or metastatic form of gestational trophoblastic disease

k. Form of gestational trophoblastic disease resulting from abnormal fertilization, in which there is proliferation of swollen chorionic villi; also called a molar pregnancy

l. Excessive vomiting. Hyperemesis during pregnancy is sometimes called hyperemesis gravidarum.

19. _____ subchorionic hemorrhage

20. _____ hyperemesis

21. _____ theca lutein cysts

22. _____ bradycardia

23. _____ miscarriage

24. _____ subchorionic hematoma

25. _____ blighted ovum

26. _____ incomplete abortion

27. _____ molar pregnancy

m. Excessive activity of the thyroid
n. Spontaneous abortion in which some products of conception remain in the uterus
o. Failed early pregnancy which is in the process of being expelled from the uterus
p. Spontaneous failure and expulsion of an early pregnancy
q. Early failed pregnancy that remains in the uterus
r. Hydatidiform mole
s. Abnormal fertilization resulting in one maternal and two paternal sets of chromosomes (triploidy), leading to the development of an abnormal fetus and placenta
t. Inadequate absorption of oxygen and/or inadequate expulsion of carbon dioxide
u. Crescent-shaped sonolucent collection of blood between the gestational sac and uterine wall
v. Subchorionic hemorrhage
w. Abnormally rapid heart rate
x. Vaginal bleeding in a pregnancy of <20 weeks; may be accompanied by pain or cramping
y. Large, often bilateral ovarian cysts, the formation of which is usually stimulated by excessive levels of circulating hCG
z. Pregnancy-induced hypertension, proteinuria, edema, and headache (preeclampsia), which may progress to the development of seizures (eclampsia)
aa. Having three copies of each chromosome

CHAPTER REVIEW

Multiple Choice

Complete each question by circling the best answer.

1. Uterine size estimation by physical examination, to determine pregnancy age, may be inaccurate owing to all except:
   a. uterine fibroids
   b. maternal obesity
   c. surgical scars
   d. parity

2. What laboratory value is useful when a smaller than expected gestational sac is seen with ultrasound?
   a. PAPP-A
   b. hCG
   c. Progesterone
   d. Estrogen

3. Early-onset intrauterine growth restriction is defined as crown–rump length at least _____ standard deviations below the mean for the expected gestational age.
   a. one
   b. two
   c. three
   d. four

4. Spontaneous pregnancy loss before 20 weeks (of clinically recognized gestations) is as high as:
   a. 30%
   b. 20%
   c. 10% to 20%
   d. 5%

5. A pregnancy less than 20 weeks with vaginal bleeding is termed:
   a. threatened abortion
   b. inevitable abortion
   c. miscarriage
   d. hemorrhagic conceptus

6. A gestational sac without an embryo or yolk scan with a mean sac diameter greater than _____ (EV) *generally* predicts pregnancy failure.
   a. 10 mm
   b. 1.5 cm
   c. 2.0 cm
   d. 25 mm

7. Select the yolk sac with the healthiest characteristics.
   a. Oblong
   b. Round
   c. Less than two standard deviations below the mean yolk sac diameter for gestational age
   d. More than two standard deviations above the mean yolk sac diameter for a given gestational age

8. Pregnancy failure is most likely to occur when the fetal heart rate is:
   a. 150 bpm at 8 weeks
   b. greater than or equal to 155 bpm at 6.3 to 7 weeks
   c. 120 to 130 bpm at 9 weeks
   d. less than 110 bpm at 6.3 to 7 weeks

9. Select the statement which does not indicate probable embryonic demise.
   a. 6-mm embryo without cardiac activity
   b. No double bleb sign with a less than 5-mm embryo
   c. No cardiac activity with a less than 5-mm embryo and a double bleb sign
   d. Enlarged amniotic sac with less than 5-mm embryo

10. The risk of spontaneous miscarriage, preeclampsia, placental abnormalities, or preterm delivery is increased by crescent-shaped sonolucent fluid between the gestational sac and the uterine wall as is called:
    a. chorionic hemorrhage
    b. subchorionic hematoma
    c. retroplacental bleed
    d. subamniotic hemorrhage

11. A complete hydatidiform mole usually results in:
    a. large-for-dates uterus and vaginal bleeding
    b. a triploid pregnancy with 69 chromosomes
    c. vaginal bleeding and a small-for-dates or normal-sized uterus
    d. a thick, hydropic placenta

12. Select the measurement not usually included in a first-trimester screening for assessing risk in a chromosomally abnormal fetus.
    a. CRL
    b. NT
    c. MSD
    d. Ductus venosus Doppler velocimetry

13. Hydatidiform moles are caused by:
    a. preeclampsia
    b. abnormal fertilization
    c. malignant neoplasms
    d. papillomavirus infection prior to pregnancy

14. Select the correct sonographic appearance for impending abortion.
    a. Early empty gestational sac
    b. Crescent-shaped fluid collection between the gestational sac and uterus
    c. Oval-shaped gestational sac
    d. Empty low-lying gestational sac, open cervix

15. Theca lutein cysts are usually stimulated by excessive levels of hCG and are related to:
    a. blighted ovum
    b. fetal aneuploidy
    c. complete molar pregnancy
    d. neoplasia

16. The recommended first-trimester screening tests for assessing the risk of carrying a chromosomally abnormal embryo include all except:
    a. measuring crown–rump length
    b. measuring nuchal translucency
    c. measuring fetal heart rate
    d. testing maternal serum biochemistry levels

17. Select a first-trimester fetal central nervous system abnormality.
    a. Dandy-Walker malformation
    b. Dysplastic kidney
    c. Ectopia cordis
    d. Gastroschisis

Fill-in-the-Blank

1. When the uterus is smaller than expected, ultrasound is used to rule out incorrect dates, early pregnancy failure, or _____ pregnancy.

2. In women with vaginal _____ or _____, the risk of pregnancy loss increases.

3. Genetic abnormalities cause _____ of pregnancy failure.

4. A patient with an anembryonic pregnancy or embryo demise that has not yet been expelled from the uterus is labeled as a _____ or _____.

5. A blighted ovum is also called a(n) _____.

6. Visualization of an amnion without sonographic evidence of an embryo is called _____.

7. Routine obstetric ultrasound done between approximately 6 and 12 weeks divulging a normal singleton fetus, demonstrates a miscarriage rate of _____.

8. An embryo measuring _____ or greater should demonstrate cardiac activity.

9. A failed early pregnancy that is in the process of being expelled from the uterus is called _____.

10. Uterine fibroids may be associated with preterm _____, premature _____ of membranes, and fetal _____.

11. Enlarged ovaries are frequently seen during complete molar pregnancy as a result of elevated _____ levels.

12. Molar pregnancy has the ability to develop into _____.

13. Holoprosencephaly is a _____ system abnormality.

14. A patient diagnosed with molar pregnancy should have a weekly blood test for _____ consecutive weeks until her hCG level returns to normal.

15. Toxemia of pregnancy presents as pregnancy-induced hypertension, proteinuria, edema, and headache (preeclampsia) and may progress to _____ (_____).

Short Answer

1. Explain how fibroids affect a pregnancy.

2. Discuss the importance of diagnosing molar pregnancy as early as possible. Explain effective treatment protocols for the condition.

3. Compare and explain the difference between first-trimester hydatidiform mole with the second-trimester hydatidiform mole.

4. Define incomplete abortion, missed abortion, inevitable abortion, and threatened abortion. Describe their ultrasound appearance.

IMAGE EVALUATION/PATHOLOGY

Review the images and answer the following questions.

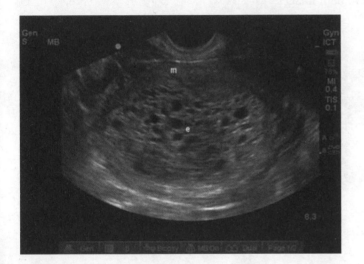

1. Explain this image of uterine contents in a 10-week gestation with reported bleeding.

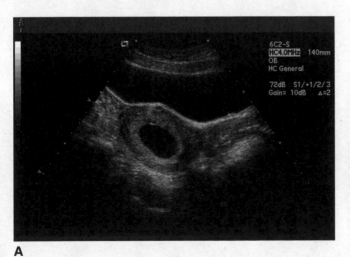

A

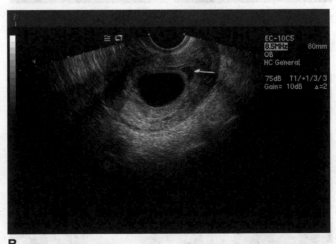

B

2. Discuss image A and image B. What is the arrow directed to in image B?

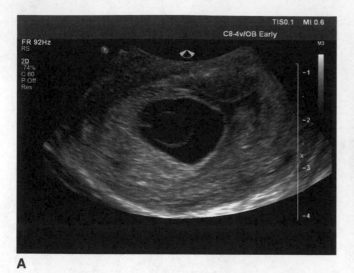

A

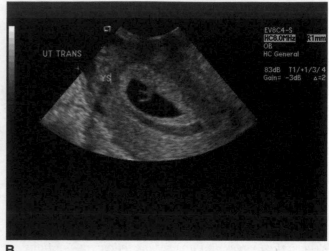

B

3. Discuss image A and image B. Explain structures seen in both images.

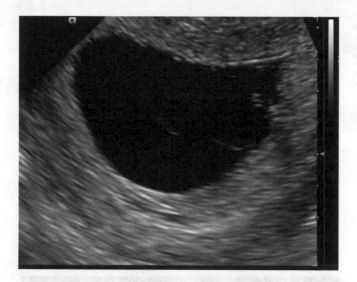

4. State the correct diagnosis for this pregnancy.

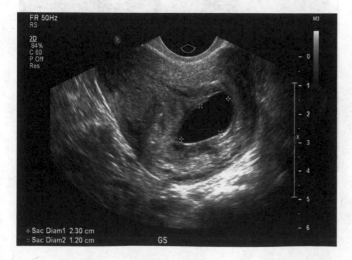

5. State the correct diagnosis for this pregnancy.

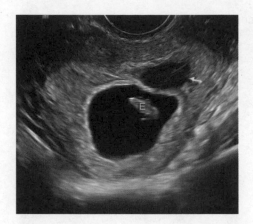

6. What is the arrow pointing toward?

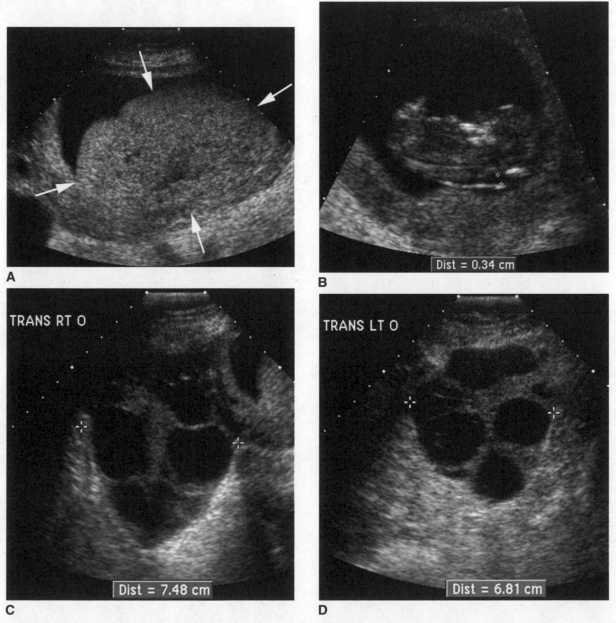

A

B

Dist = 0.34 cm

TRANS RT O

Dist = 7.48 cm

C

TRANS LT O

Dist = 6.81 cm

D

7. Diagnose this pregnancy. There is no fetal cardiac activity.

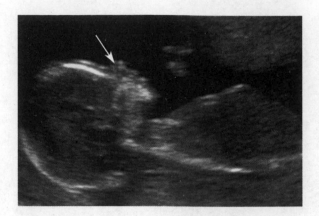

8. Diagnose the image using the arrow as a hint.

CHAPTER 19

Sonographic Assessment of the Ectopic Pregnancy

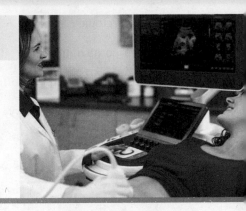

REVIEW OF GLOSSARY TERMS

Matching

Match the key terms with their definitions.

KEY TERMS

1. _____ intramural pregnancy

2. _____ double decidual sac sign

3. _____ pregnancy of unknown location (PUL)

4. _____ abdominal pregnancy

5. _____ intrauterine contraceptive device (IUD)

6. _____ sliding sac sign

7. _____ heterotopic pregnancy

8. _____ beta human chorionic gonadotropin (beta-hCG)

9. _____ hypovolemic shock

10. _____ tubal ring sign

11. _____ cervical pregnancy

12. _____ Morison pouch

13. _____ pelvic inflammatory disease (PID)

14. _____ assisted reproductive techniques (ARTs)

15. _____ ovarian pregnancy

16. _____ in vitro fertilization (IVF)

17. _____ interstitial pregnancy

DEFINITIONS

a. Gestation located within the intraperitoneal cavity, apart from tubal, ovarian, or intralegamentous sites

b. A number of techniques used to aid fertilization; including in vitro fertilization (IVF), intracytoplasmic sperm insertion (ICSI), follicle aspiration, sperm injection, assisted follicular rupture (FASIAR)

c. Glycoprotein hormone produced in pregnancy that is made by the developing embryo soon after conception and later by the placenta

d. Gestation located within the endocervical canal

e. Gestation located within a rudimentary uterine horn or one horn of a bicornuate or septated uterus or a gestation located within a rudimentary horn of a uterus with a Müllerian anomaly

f. Two concentric hyperechoic rings (representing the echogenic base of the endometrium and the decidua capsularis/chorion laeve) surrounding the anechoic gestational sac in a normal intrauterine pregnancy

g. Implantation of a fertilized ovum in any area outside of the endometrial cavity

h. Concomitant intrauterine pregnancy and ectopic pregnancy

i. Life-threatening condition owing to a decrease in blood volume

j. Gestation located in the intramyometrial segment of the fallopian tube

k. Gestation located within the myometrium of the uterus

l. Form of birth control; small, plastic or copper, usually T-shaped device with a string attached to the end that is inserted into the uterus

m. Laboratory procedure in which sperm are placed with an unfertilized egg in a petri dish to achieve fertilization; the embryo is then transferred into the uterus to begin a pregnancy or cryopreserved for future use

18. _____ ectopic pregnancy

19. _____ cornual pregnancy

20. _____ discriminatory cutoff

21. _____ eccentric pregnancy

n. Level of beta-hCG at which a normal intrauterine pregnancy can be seen with sonography

o. Gestation located with the superior-lateral aspect of the endometrial cavity

p. Infection of the female reproductive tract that results from microorganisms transmitted especially during sexual intercourse or by other means such as during surgery, abortion, or parturition

q. Pregnancy in which no signs of an intrauterine pregnancy or ectopic pregnancy are seen by sonography

r. When gentle pressure from the transducer moves the gestational sac

s. Hyperechoic ring of trophoblastic tissue that surrounds an extrauterine gestational sac

t. Hepatorenal recess; deep recess of the peritoneal cavity on the right side extending upward between the liver and the kidney; gravity-dependent portion of the peritoneal cavity when in the supine position

u. Gestation located within the ovary

ANATOMY AND PHYSIOLOGY REVIEW

Image Labeling

Complete the labels in the images that follow.

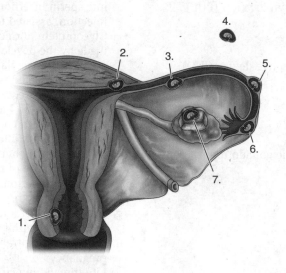

Ectopic pregnancy implantation sites

CHAPTER REVIEW

Multiple Choice

Complete each question by circling the best answer.

1. Ectopic pregnancy can be caused by:
   a. elevated beta-hCG
   b. hypovolemic shock
   c. oviduct surgical history
   d. irregular sperm motility

2. Signs of tubal rupture may include all but:
   a. hypotension
   b. rebound tenderness
   c. tachycardia
   d. UTI

3. When are ectopic pregnancies usually diagnosed?
   a. 2 to 4 weeks
   b. 4 to 8 weeks
   c. 6 to 10 weeks
   d. 8 to 12 weeks

4. Beta-hCG levels should approximately double every _____ hours:
   a. 48
   b. 36
   c. 24
   d. 12

5. At what level of beta-hCG concentration should a normal intrauterine pregnancy be seen?
   a. 3.000 to 10,000 U/mL
   b. 1,500 to 2,500 mIU/mL
   c. 500 to 1,000 mIU/L
   d. 2,000 to 3,000 mIU/mL

6. Interstitial pregnancy occurs in the:
   a. rudimentary uterine horn
   b. cervical interstitial
   c. cornua
   d. intramyometrial segment of the fallopian tube

7. Ectopic pregnancy most often implant in the:
   a. fallopian tube
   b. ovary
   c. cornua
   d. cervix

8. Even though it is implanted within the uterine cavity, a cornual pregnancy is classified as an ectopic pregnancy because of its propensity to rupture in the:
   a. early first trimester, weeks 4 to 9
   b. late first trimester, weeks 9 to 13
   c. second trimester
   d. third trimester

9. Cervical pregnancy is rare and linked to all of the following except:
   a. previous curettage
   b. ovulation induction techniques
   c. endometriosis
   d. IUD use

10. Procedures that cause an injury to the myometrium, including curettage, hysteroscopy, myomectomy, metroplasty, and cesarean section can be the cause for _____ pregnancy.
    a. infundibular
    b. interstitial
    c. heterotopic
    d. intramural

11. Heterotopic pregnancy means pregnancy:
    a. outside the uterus
    b. eccentric in the uterus
    c. simultaneously positioned intrauterine and extrauterine
    d. with bleeding

12. What beta-hCG levels are necessary to visualize an IUP using transabdominal approach?
    a. 2,500 mU/L
    b. 4,000 IU/m
    c. 6,500 mIU/mL
    d. 8,500 mIU/mL

13. Which ectopic pregnancy location can support a pregnancy the longest before detection?
    a. Abdominal
    b. Ovarian
    c. Cervical
    d. Intramural

14. A pseudosac:
    a. is a true gestational sac positioned low in the uterine cavity
    b. is a fluid collection caused by bleeding from the decidualized endometrium
    c. abuts the endometrial canal
    d. has a double decidual sac sign

15. Cervical pregnancy frequently presents on ultrasound as a(n) _____ shaped uterus:
    a. oval
    b. cylindrical
    c. "T"
    d. hourglass

16. A sonographic technique that can assist in determining if a gestation is an abortion in progress versus a cervical pregnancy or cesarean scar pregnancy is:
    a. graded compression
    b. the abdominal approach
    c. color Doppler
    d. low resistive index

17. A ruptured tubal pregnancy presents as a:
    a. complex mass-like area representing hemorrhage and free fluid
    b. circumscribed mass
    c. solid heterogeneous mass with irregular borders
    d. hypoechoic cyst with nodular internal foci

18. An aborting gestational sac will appear _____ with color Doppler.
    a. poorly perfused
    b. avascular
    c. well perfused
    d. as a pseudosac

19. If ultrasound is equivocal in the diagnosis of ectopic pregnancy, _____ may be used for diagnosis.
    a. laparoscopy
    b. laparotomy
    c. culdocentesis
    d. curettage

20. What imaging method is considered the "gold standard" for diagnosing and locating an abdominal ectopic pregnancy?
    a. TV ultrasound
    b. TA ultrasound
    c. CT
    d. MRI

Fill-in-the-Blank

1. About _____ of all pregnancies in the U.S. are ectopic.

2. The pathway from the uterine cavity to the peritoneal cavity is through the _____.

3. Beta-hCG levels increase and then plateau at approximately _____ weeks.

4. Repeated or _____ beta-hCG levels are necessary to detect an increase, decrease, or leveling of the hormone.

5. When the beta-hCG level is below the discriminatory cutoff and an IUP is not visualized, this could indicate an early _____, a spontaneous abortion, or an _____ pregnancy.

6. Ectopic pregnancy symptoms usually present as vaginal _____, pelvic _____, and palpable _____.

7. _____ pain is the most frequent symptom seen with heterotopic pregnancy.

8. Ovarian _____ surrounds an ovarian pregnancy.

9. Symptoms of general malaise, nausea, vomiting, vaginal bleeding, and painful fetal movements are associated with _____ ectopic pregnancy.

10. Transvaginal sonography should demonstrate a fetal pole with cardiac motion at _____ weeks gestation.

11. Sonographic evaluation of ectopic pregnancy should include the _____ recess and paracolic _____ to evaluate for the extent of free fluid.

12. An endometrial stripe thickness less than _____ mm suggests an abnormal or ectopic pregnancy.

13. Three criteria for interstitial pregnancy are _____ uterine cavity, gestational sac greater than _____ cm from the most lateral point of the endometrial cavity, and gestational sac surrounded by a thin _____ layer.

14. The sliding sac sign suggests an _____ in progress.

15. The yolk sac should be visualized by _____ weeks' gestation.

16. The area most likely to collect fluid in the right abdomen between the liver and kidney is called _____.

17. Color Doppler presents as a _____ around a viable ectopic pregnancy.

18. In the setting of an ectopic pregnancy, the uterus may appear _____.

19. MTX, known as _____, interferes with cell _____ and is used to manage ectopic pregnancy in a _____ manner.

20. Findings on physical examination of a pregnant female vary with the hemodynamic condition of the patient; hypotension, tachycardia, shoulder pain from diaphragmatic irritation, significant abdominal pain, rebound tenderness and guarding, hypovolemic shock, or even diminished pain may all be signs of _____ and/or _____.

Short Answer

1. List reasons that fertilized ovum may have difficulty transporting to the endometrial cavity.

2. Describe the expected appearance of an extrauterine pregnancy.

3. A 23-year-old G2 P1 presents to the emergency department with right adnexal pain. Routine laboratory testing documented pregnancy and a normal WBC. Ultrasound was ordered and demonstrated a normal, empty uterine cavity and the right ovary to have what appeared to be an echogenic corpus luteum cyst with a wide echogenic ring demonstrating color flow. Make a diagnosis.

4. Explain the time frame for visualization of the yolk sac, cardiac activity, and double decidual sac sign.

IMAGE EVALUATION/PATHOLOGY

Review the images and answer the following questions.

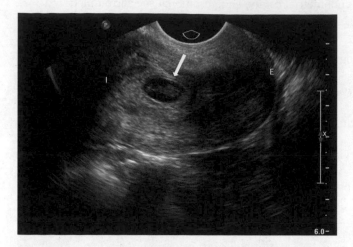

1. State the anatomy the arrow is directed at and name the pelvic structure.

2. What is the location of the pregnancy in the image on question #1?

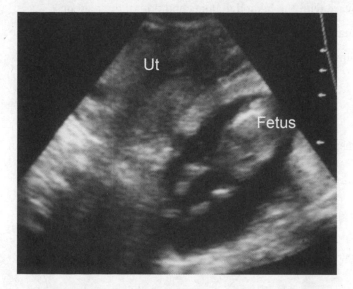

3. What ultrasound imaging method collected the image? State the location of the ectopic pregnancy.

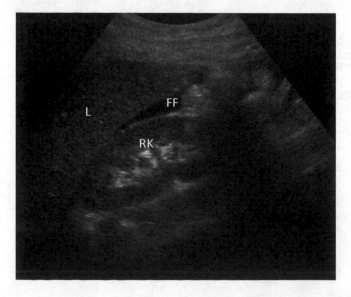

4. Explain a probable reason for free fluid in this patient with a known ectopic ruptured tubal pregnancy. Name the region of the fluid collection.

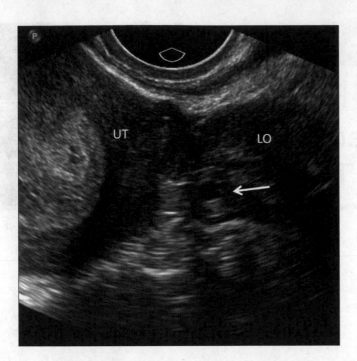

5. Label the structure depicted by the arrow in this transverse transvaginal image.

CHAPTER 20

Assessment of Fetal Age and Size in the Second and Third Trimester

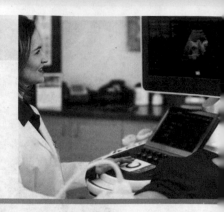

REVIEW OF GLOSSARY TERMS

Matching

Match the key terms with their definitions.

KEY TERMS

1. _____ macrosomia

2. _____ cephalic index (CI)

3. _____ occipito-frontal diameter (OFD)

4. _____ predictive value

5. _____ axial resolution

DEFINITIONS

a. Minimum distance between two bright echoes along the path of the ultrasound beam which is half the spatial pulse length
b. Measurement from the frontal to the occipital obtained at the same level as the BPD
c. Precision rate of the probability of disease
d. Ratio of the BPD to the OFD
e. Fetus over 4,000 g (8 pounds, 13 ounces)

CHAPTER REVIEW

Multiple Choice

Complete each question by circling the best answer.

1. The fetal expected birth date is known as the EDC or:
   a. GA
   b. EDD
   c. GA
   d. LMP

2. The most accurate fetal measurement in the second and third trimesters can be obtained from:
   a. the BPD
   b. the AC and FL
   c. the HC
   d. multiple parameters

3. Which phase of pregnancy provides the most accurate dating?
   a. Early embryo measurements
   b. Early second trimester, 16 to 18 weeks
   c. Late second trimester, 25 to 26 weeks
   d. Early third trimester, 28 to 29 weeks

4. The preferred measurement method for fetal growth is:
   a. one single measurement
   b. BPD, FL, AC, HL, HC
   c. average of multiple measurements, three or more
   d. HC, AC, FL

5. The normal duration of pregnancy is:
   a. 40 weeks from ovulation
   b. 40 weeks from the LMP
   c. conception date plus 40 weeks
   d. GA plus 4 weeks

6. Hadlock and coworkers and Ott determined the accurate indicator of fetal age is determined by:
   a. single fetal parameter average age
   b. FPA
   c. multiple fetal parameter average age
   d. femoral diaphysis length

7. The earliest successful BPD measurement can usually be secured at week:
   a. 10
   b. 12
   c. 16
   d. 20

8. If the cerebellum is seen in a BPD measurement, the plane is ____ in the posterior portion of the image.
   a. too lateral
   b. correct
   c. too high
   d. too low

9. The most common and routine measurements to assess the fetal growth and well-being are:
   a. HL, FL, HC, and AC
   b. FL, HC, AC, and OD
   c. BPD, HC, AC, and FL
   d. BPD, AC, HC, and MFP

10. Select a fetal characteristic that is not a late gestational individuation.
    a. elongated fetus
    b. dolichocephaly
    c. thin fetus
    d. bradycardia

11. What structures are seen in an accurate BPD measurement?
    a. Complete oval calvarium, sphenoid and petrous bones
    b. Thalamus, cavum magnum
    c. Complete oval calvarium with the cerebellum demonstrated
    d. Orbital, base X, occipital

12. To estimate an accurate fetal age, the BPD measurement should be obtained before:
    a. 29 weeks
    b. 31 weeks
    c. 33 weeks
    d. 35 weeks

13. An HC measurement should be obtained:
    a. using the inner edge of the calvarium at the level of the BPD
    b. using the outer edge of the calvarium at the level of the BPD
    c. using the outer edge of the calvarium at the level of the cerebellum
    d. at the level of the occipital circumference

14. Select the correct CI formula:
    a. $(D1 + D2) \times 1.57$
    b. $BPD/FOD \times 100$
    c. $89\%/OD \times (d_1 - d_2)$
    d. $FOD/BPD \times 100$

15. Platycephaly is:
    a. premature closure of the cranial sutures
    b. flattening of the forehead, causing skull widening
    c. a type of coneheadedness
    d. shortening of the vertical dimension of the skull

16. The most exact of the orbit measurements is the:
    a. BOD
    b. OOD
    c. IOD
    d. IGE

17. All of the following are fetal long bones except:
    a. tibia
    b. humerus
    c. metacarpal
    d. ulna

18. Fetal weight by ultrasound is frequently requested to rule out all except:
    a. macrosomia
    b. BPP
    c. IUGR
    d. possible low birth weight

19. If the umbilical/portal junction is not visualized while attempting an AC measurement, use the level of the fetal:
    a. stomach
    b. kidneys
    c. adrenals
    d. cord insertion

20. Preferred technique for measuring the fetal abdomen and head circumference is:
    a. manual tracing
    b. ellipse
    c. inner skin line
    d. two-point

Fill-in-the-Blank

1. Two purposes for second and third trimester measurements of a fetus are estimating _____ and determining the size and development.

2. Differences in fetal growth parameters can be caused by maternal _____, _____, and genetics.

3. Normally conception takes place about _____ weeks after the LMP.

4. Molding and normal morphologic variations of the fetal head have a great effect on the accuracy of the _____ measurement in assessing age.

5. Exclude the _____ of the scalp when measuring from the leading edge of the parietal bone for a BPD measurement.

6. When taking fetal measurements, always use the transducer and focal range that provide the _____ resolution.

7. Macrosomia equates to a fetus over _____ g.

8. If the fetal head is very low in the pelvis, a(n) _____ transducer may allow accurate BPD measurements.

9. The head circumference should be measured on the same image used for the _____ measurement.

10. The more measurements obtained and averaged during a fetal ultrasound, the more _____ the fetal age estimate.

11. MFP (_____) is the average gestational age determined by four common measurements of the fetus.

12. A measurement of the HC using the perimeter tracing method should be made around the _____ edge of the calvarium.

13. A fetus with a long and narrow head is called _____.

14. Cerebellar size is generally unaffected by fetal _____ disturbances and is independent of the shape of the _____.

15. A correct AC measurement demonstrates the _____ vein junction with the _____ vein perpendicular to the _____.

16. A structure within the cranium that maintains a relationship to fetal growth throughout pregnancy is the

    _____.

17. Common fetal body ratios are _____, _____, and _____.

18. The recommended technique to obtaining an accurate AC is to first locate the long axis of the _____.

19. The outer _____ line must be included in the abdominal circumference so that AC is not

    underestimated.

20. The femur measurement can be reliably used after _____ weeks gestation.

Short Answer

1. Ann has a history of oligomenorrhea. She is G3 P2. Her first pregnancy delivered close to her EDD and the second delivered 3 weeks early owing to incompetent cervix. Explain reasons why accurate fetal dating is important for this pregnancy, as well as all pregnancies.

2. Discuss reasons the BPD measurement can be inaccurate.

3. Explain dolichocephaly and brachycephaly and their relationship to CI.

4. A student sonographer continually obtained FL measurements 6 to 11 days longer than the other fetal parameters on the second- and third-trimester fetal examinations. What is a probable explanation? Discuss the correct femur measurement technique.

IMAGE EVALUATION/PATHOLOGY

Review the images and answer the following questions.

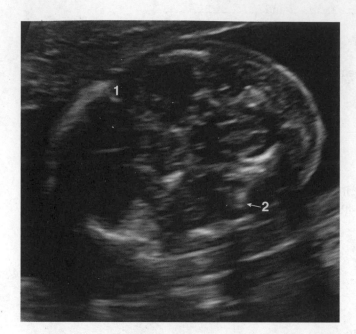

1. Name the structure/bones seen in this image.

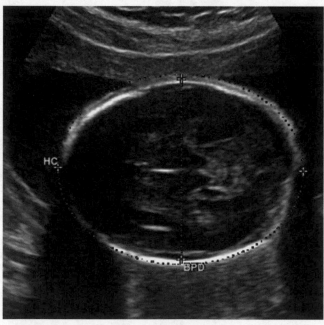

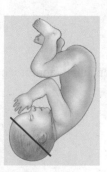

2. State the measurements obtained in the image.

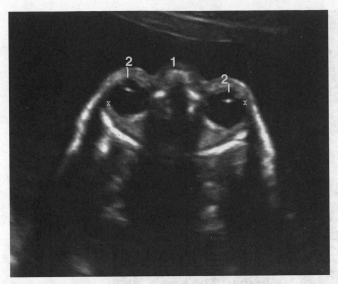
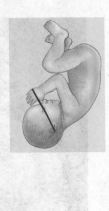

3. Label #1, #2, and explain the two x's on the image.

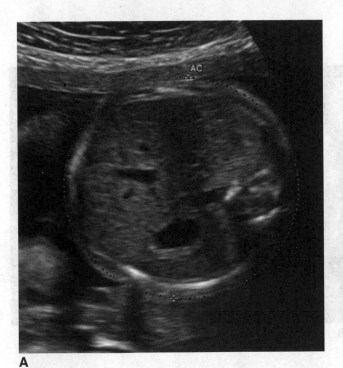
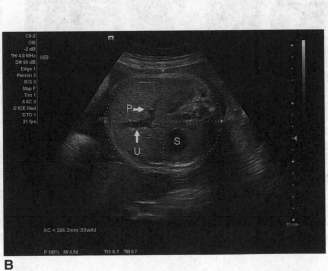

A

B

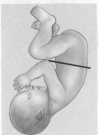

4. Identify the structure. Explain the proper way to measure it.

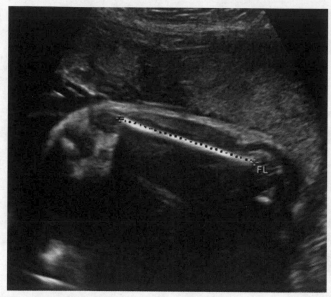

5. Identify the structure. Explain the proper way to measure it.

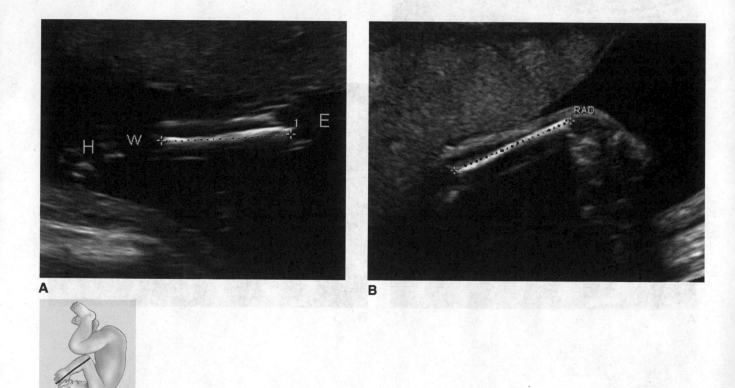

A

B

6. Label images A and B.

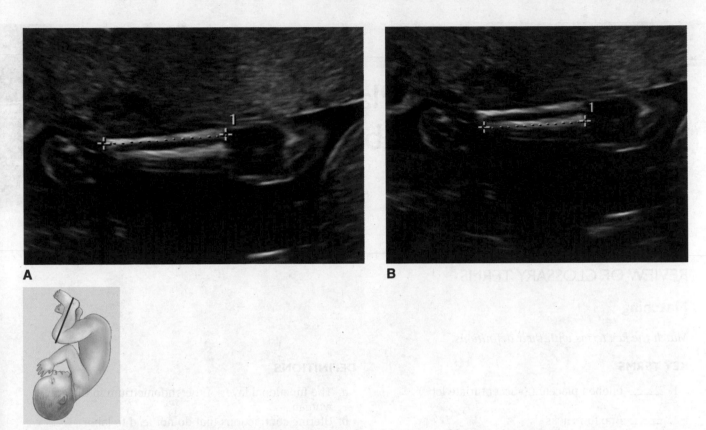

A

B

7. Name the measured lower extremity bone in image A, then the measured bone in image B.

Hint: Note the thickness of each bone.

CHAPTER 21

Normal Placenta and Umbilical Cord

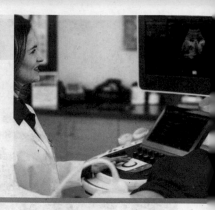

REVIEW OF GLOSSARY TERMS

Matching

Match the key terms with their definitions.

KEY TERMS

1. _____ bilobed placenta (succenturiate lobe)

2. _____ Braxton-Hicks

3. _____ cotyledons

4. _____ decidua

5. _____ retroplacental

6. _____ Valsalva

7. _____ vernix caseosum

8. _____ Wharton jelly

DEFINITIONS

a. The functional layer of the endometrium in the gravid woman
b. Uterine contractions that do not lead to labor
c. Inhalation and suspension of breath coupled with abdominal muscle contraction to increase abdominal pressure
d. White, cheese-like coating of fetal skin
e. Extra placental lobe smaller than the placenta
f. Area between the myometrium and placenta
g. Mucous tissue surrounding the umbilical cord
h. Lobule or subdivision of the maternal placenta containing fetal vessels, chorionic villi, and the intervillous space

ANATOMY AND PHYSIOLOGY REVIEW

Image Labeling

Complete the labels in the images that follow.

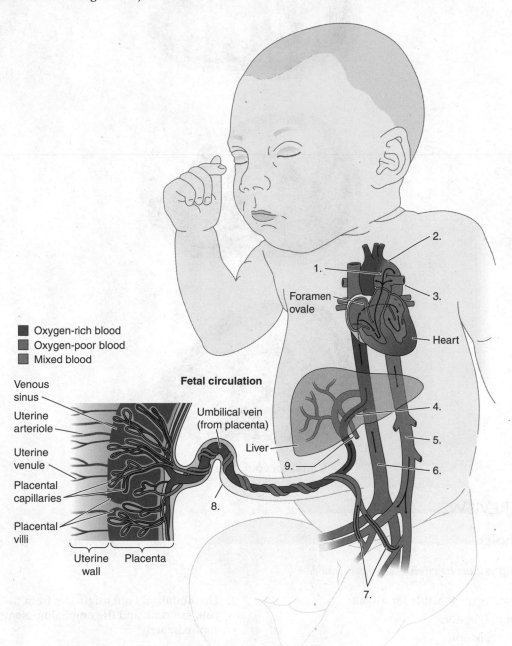

Fetal circulation

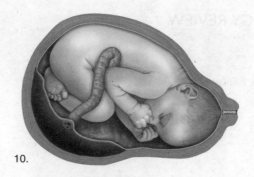

10.

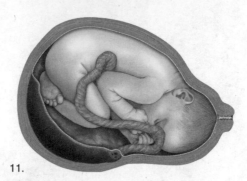

11.

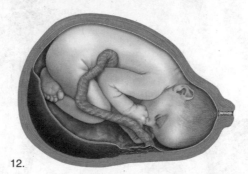

12.

Umbilical cord insertions

CHAPTER REVIEW

Multiple Choice

Complete each question by circling the best answer.

1. The placenta is responsible for all but:
   a. hormonal functions
   b. nutritive functions
   c. respiratory functions
   d. excretory functions

2. Vascular resistance changes in the umbilical cord can be caused by all except:
   a. umbilical cord compression
   b. maternal hypotension
   c. placental tumor
   d. maternal diabetes

3. The umbilical cord originates from fusion of the yolk sac stalk and the omphalomesenteric duct at approximately:
   a. 7 weeks gestation
   b. 6 weeks gestation
   c. 5 weeks gestation
   d. 4 weeks gestation

4. The maternal side of the placenta:
   a. is homogeneous
   b. is made of approximately 20 cotyledons
   c. is bordered by amnion
   d. attaches to the chorionic plate

5. The umbilical cord consists of:
   a. two veins, an artery, and a layer of amnion
   b. two veins, an artery, and surrounding mucoid epithelial tissue
   c. two arteries, a vein, and a layer of chorion
   d. two arteries, a vein, and Wharton jelly

6. The normal at term umbilical cord length is approximately:
   a. 40 to 45 cm
   b. 44 to 52 cm
   c. 52 to 61 cm
   d. 75 cm

7. The normal term placenta weighs between:
   a. 250 and 320 g
   b. 330 and 450 g
   c. 480 and 600 g
   d. 570 and 660 g

8. A normal placental thickness at 24 weeks gestation is less than:
   a. 2 cm
   b. 3 cm
   c. 4 cm
   d. 5 cm

9. Placental calcification may be caused by all except:
   a. lung maturity
   b. maternal smoking
   c. parity
   d. season of the year

10. A normal mean circumference of the term umbilical cord is:
    a. 3.8 cm
    b. 2.8 cm
    c. 4.0 cm
    d. 2.5 cm

Fill-in-the-Blank

1. More than _____ of placentas show macroscopic calcification after _____ weeks.

2. _____ carry deoxygenated blood from the fetus to the placenta. The _____ returns blood back to the fetus from the placenta.

3. The umbilical _____ are longer than the _____ and wind around it.

4. The use of _____ should make visualization of the umbilical cord insertion into the placenta easily identifiable.

5. An eccentric cord insertion (near the margin) to the placenta is called _____.

6. Maternal disease can affect the size, vascularization, and _____ of the placenta.

7. The vascular channels within the placenta are part of a _____-impedance system.

8. A _____ MHz transducer is adequate for most routine imaging of the placenta.

9. A(n) _____ bladder can cause a false-positive appearance of placenta previa.

10. When scanning the placenta, the beam should be _____ to the chorionic plate, especially when measuring thickness.

11. An accessory placental lobe is also known as a _____ lobe.

12. Placental texture changes from an _____ focal thickening of the wall of the gestational sac early in pregnancy to the fine, granular, _____ texture seen from the end of the first trimester.

13. The umbilical artery has a _____-resistance, _____ diastolic blood flow characteristic in the normal placenta.

14. A late third-trimester placenta may exhibit cystic areas located centrally within clearly delineated lobes which may represent areas of _____.

15. The nutrient exchange between the fetus and the mother occurs within the _____ in the placenta.

IMAGE EVALUATION/PATHOLOGY

Review the images and answer the following questions.

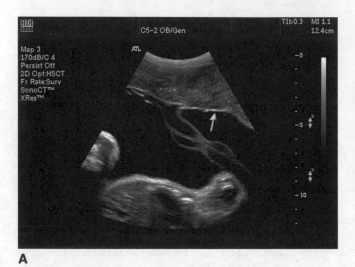

A

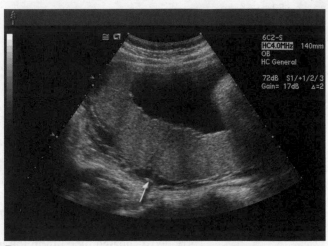

B

1. State the anatomy the arrows are directed at in images A and B.

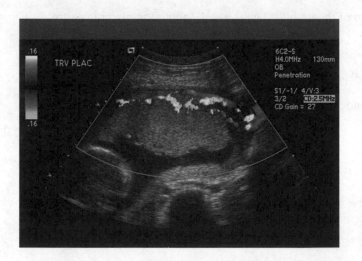

2. Explain the bright white patterns in the image. Grade the placenta.

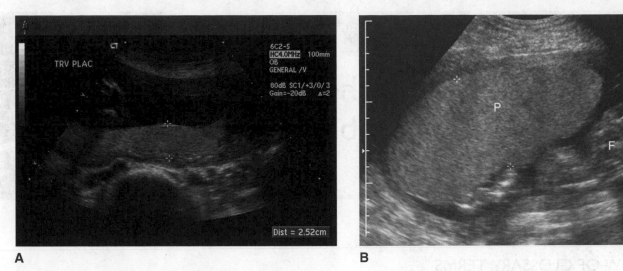

A   **B**

3. Does the placental thickness measurement in the image include the retroplacental thickness? Should it? Does the thickness appear normal?

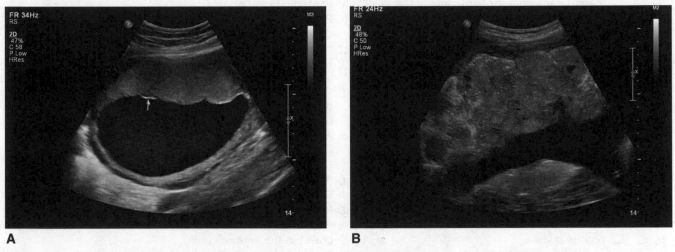

A   **B**

4. Grade the placenta and describe the left image A. Grade the placenta and describe the right image B.

CHAPTER 22

Abnormalities of the Placenta and Umbilical Cord

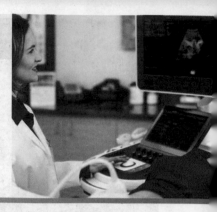

REVIEW OF GLOSSARY TERMS

Matching

Match the key terms with their definitions.

KEY TERMS

1. _____ marginal insertion or battledore placenta

2. _____ umbilical coiling index (UCI)

3. _____ gastroschisis

4. _____ umbilical hernia

5. _____ extrachorial placenta

6. _____ thrombosis

7. _____ body stalk anomaly

8. _____ synechiae (Asherman syndrome)

9. _____ venous lakes

10. _____ limb–body wall complex

11. _____ umbilical cord

12. _____ false knot

13. _____ true knot

14. _____ Breus mole

15. _____ bilobed placenta

16. _____ omphalocele

17. _____ aneurysm

18. _____ placentomegaly

DEFINITIONS

a. Focal dilatation of an artery

b. Placenta where the lobes are nearly equal in size and the cord inserts into the chorionic bridge of tissue that connects the two lobes

c. Fatal condition associated with multiple congenital anomalies and absence of the umbilical cord

d. Very rare condition where there is massive subchorionic thrombosis of the placenta secondary to extreme venous obstruction

e. Attachment of the placental membranes to the fetal surface of the placenta rather than to the underlying villous placental margin

f. Bending, twisting, and bulging of the umbilical cord vessels mimicking a knot in the umbilical cord

g. Periumbilical abdominal wall defect, typically to the right of normal cord insertion that allows for free-floating bowel in the amniotic fluid

h. Condition characterized by multiple complex fetal anomalies and a short umbilical cord

i. Occurs when the umbilical cord inserts at the placental margin

j. Central anterior abdominal wall defect at the site of cord insertion into the fetal abdomen that results in abdominal organs protruding outside the abdominal cavity but contained by a covering membrane consisting of peritoneum, Wharton jelly, and amnion

k. Term that refers to a thickened or hydropic placenta

l. Linear, extra amniotic tissue that projects into the amniotic cavity with no restriction of fetal movement

m. Intraplacental area of hemorrhage and clot

n. Result of fetus passing through a loop or loops of umbilical cord creating one or more knots in the cord

o. Failure of the normal physiologic gut herniation to regress into the abdomen, resulting in a small amount of bowel protruding into the base of the umbilical cord

p. Vascular structure connecting the fetus and placenta that normally contains two arteries and one vein surrounded by Wharton jelly

q. Method of assessing the degree of umbilical cord coiling, defined as the number of complete coils per centimeter length of cord

r. Tubular, anechoic structures found beneath the chorionic plate that correspond to blood-filled spaces found at delivery

ANATOMY AND PHYSIOLOGY REVIEW

Image Labeling

Complete the labels in the images that follow.

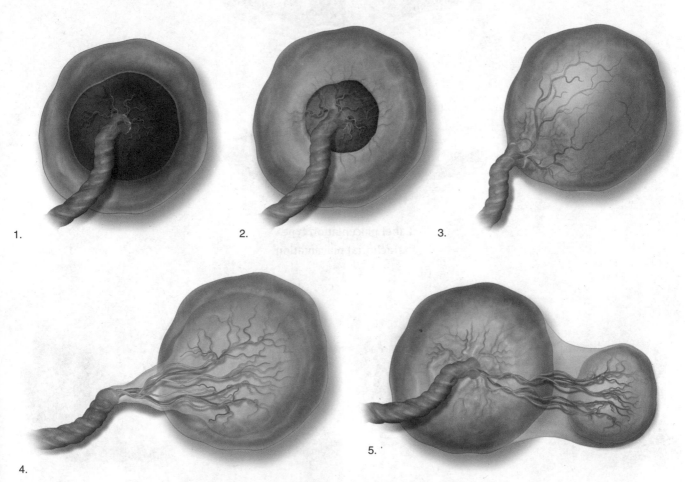

1.

2.

3.

4.

5.

Label placenta type.
Abnormalities of umbilical cord or membrane insertion into the placenta

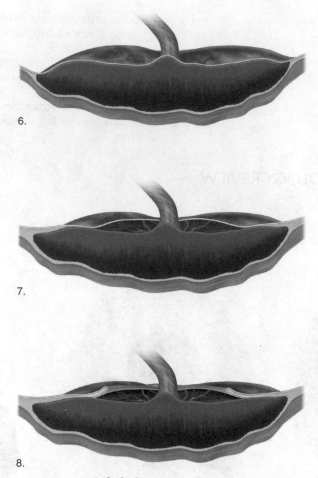

6.

7.

8.

Label placentation type.
Extrachorial placentation

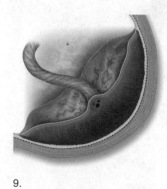

9.

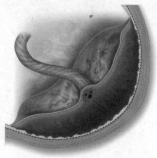

10.

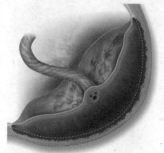

11.

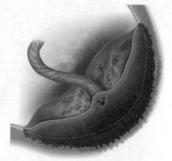

12.

Label type of accreta.
Placenta accreta spectrum classification

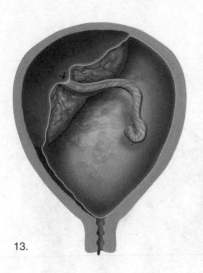

13.

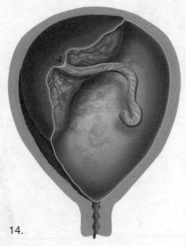

14.

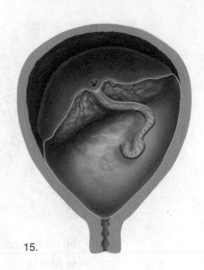

15.

Label type of abruption.

Abruptio placentae

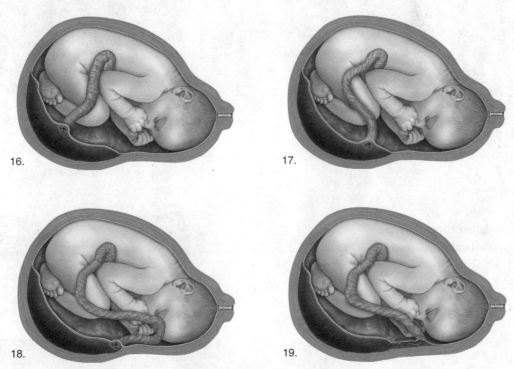

16.

17.

18.

19.

Label type of cord insertion.

Placental cord insertion

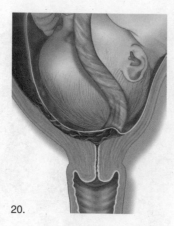

20.

Label the cord type.
Vasa previa

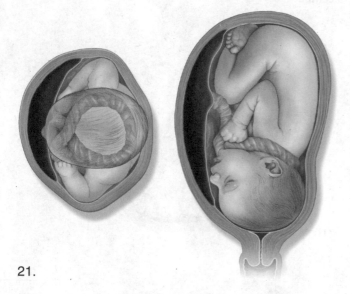

21.

Label the cord type.
Umbilical cord

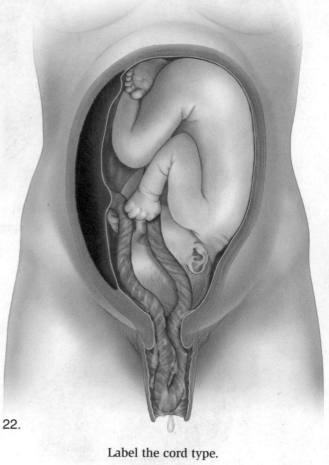

22.

Label the cord type.
Umbilical cord

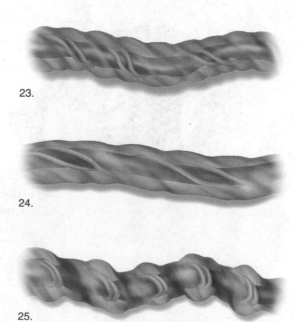

23.

24.

25.

Label the coil type.
Umbilical cord

CHAPTER REVIEW

Multiple Choice

Complete each question by circling the best answer.

1. Placental hydrops produces a:
   a. thin placenta with venous lakes
   b. thick placenta with a "ground-glass appearance"
   c. annular placenta with irregular contour
   d. membranacea placenta with low resistance blood flow

2. A "jelly-like placenta" is associated with:
   a. venous lakes
   b. IUGR
   c. adjacent fibroids
   d. degeneration

3. A succenturiate placenta:
   a. has increased frequency in primigravidas
   b. is ring shaped
   c. most often have velamentous umbilical cord insertion
   d. is edematous

4. Circumvallate placental tissue is:
   a. flat and noted on approximately 20% of placentas
   b. associated with a thickened rolled chorioamniotic membrane
   c. extremely rare, 1:20,000 to 40,000 pregnancies
   d. prone to fetal macrosomia

5. Risk factors for placenta previa include all except:
   a. previous cesarean section
   b. multiple gestations
   c. previous elective abortions
   d. hypertension

6. A placenta is considered low-lying if the inferior margin is:
   a. 0.5 cm from the internal os
   b. adjacent to the internal os
   c. within 2 cm of the internal os
   d. posterior

7. The most infiltrative form of placenta accreta is:
   a. percreta
   b. accreta
   c. increta
   d. invasive

8. Attachment problems of the placenta are known as all except:
   a. morbidly adherent placenta
   b. placental attachment disorder
   c. abnormally invasive placenta
   d. infiltrative myometrial placenta

9. Placental infarction is:
   a. visualized at the fetal placental surface
   b. owing to obstructed spiral arteries
   c. multiple hemorrhages into placental lakes
   d. a factor in macrosomia

10. A benign vascular malformation of the placenta is a:
    a. teratoma
    b. septal cyst
    c. lacunae
    d. chorioangioma

11. Premature separation of all or part of the placenta from the myometrium is:
    a. hemorrhage
    b. subchorionic
    c. abruption
    d. subdural

12. Linear, extra amniotic tissue projecting into the amniotic cavity is noted often in pregnant women with a history of:
    a. uterine curettage
    b. cervical dilation
    c. multiples
    d. STDs

13. Amniotic band syndrome is a condition that:
    a. involves free-floating membrane
    b. is a result of rupture of the amnion without rupture of the chorion
    c. is not revealed in the third trimester
    d. involves the uterine septum

14. A condition of pregnancy where the trophoblastic cells produce excessive amounts of beta-human chorionic gonadotropin is:
    a. multiparity
    b. fetal entrapment
    c. molar pregnancy (hydatidiform mole)
    d. compression syndrome

15. SUA is associated with all except:
    a. cardiovascular malformations
    b. central nervous system defects
    c. musculoskeletal abnormalities
    d. skeletal dysplasia

16. PRUV, a common vascular variant, describes:
    a. a strictured right portal vein
    b. a duplicated right portal vein
    c. pancreatic right portal vein
    d. open right portal vein

17. TTTS is caused by:
    a. battledore umbilical insertion
    b. monochorionic twin pregnancies sharing a placenta with anastomoses between the umbilical vessels
    c. oligohydramnios
    d. discordant fetal size and polyhydramnios

18. Prenatal management of known umbilical pseudo and true cysts:
    a. is not necessary because resolution is imminent
    b. typically refers to MRI for evaluation
    c. involves serial ultrasound examinations
    d. displays echogenic characteristics near the placental insertion

19. Cord prolapse is defined as:
    a. a compressed umbilical cord
    b. presentation of the umbilical cord in advance of the fetal presenting part during labor and delivery
    c. excessive bending and twisting of the umbilical cord
    d. focal bulge or vascular protuberance of the umbilical cord

Fill-in-the-Blank

1. Subamniotic cysts or subamniotic hematomas result from rupture of _____ close to the umbilical cord insertion into the placenta.

2. Selective loss of placental parts and growth of other parts is known as _____.

3. The ring-shaped annular placenta is related to postpartum _____ mostly owing to poor separation.

4. Acute placental abruption hemorrhage appears highly _____ on ultrasound.

5. Choriocarcinomas appear as _____, echogenic, and _____ masses.

6. Placenta accreta is mostly located in the _____, _____ uterine segment.

7. Visualization of multiple _____ are highly suggestive of placenta accreta.

8. Multiple chorioangiomas or those larger than _____ cm are related to maternal and fetal complications.

9. Early detection of fetal anemia is possible where chorioangioma is suspected, through Doppler measurements of the _____.

10. Extremely hydropic and swollen chorionic villi are frequently related to _____.

11. Molar pregnancies have a characteristic _____ appearance with uterine cavity _____.

12. The most common reason for emergency postpartum hysterectomy is a _____.

13. A coexisting fetus with an enlarged thickened placenta revealing multiple small cystic spaces is a _____.

14. The placenta may sonographically appear thickened in some cases of IUGR, with patchy areas of _____ and abnormal texture.

15. A two-vessel umbilical cord reveals the presence of a single umbilical _____ and is sometimes associated with congenital anomalies such as cardiovascular malformations, central nervous system defects, _____ or genitourinary defects, and _____ malformations.

16. The umbilical vessel abnormality seen with conjoined twins is _____ vessels.

17. Maternal cocaine abuse leads to the fatal condition _____.

18. Velamentous insertion is more frequent in _____ gestations.

19. Compressed umbilical cords place the fetus at risk for _____ or _____ compromise.

20. A successful method of identifying a nuchal cord is imaging using _____ technology.

Short Answer

1. An obstetrical patient in her 32nd week of pregnancy presents to ultrasound for transient anterior pelvic pain. Ultrasound revealed unusual Doppler patterns at the anterior inferior uterine wall adjacent to the anterior mid-level placenta and hypoechoic regions. Discuss a diagnosis and other sonographic signs that may be demonstrated.

2. Compare placenta accreta to increta and percreta. State risk factors.

3. A 34-week G2 patient presents to the emergency department complaining of 3 hours of intense pain near her belly button. Ultrasound noted a viable fetus with no appearance of obvious distress and a normal-appearing fundal anterior placenta. Suggest a diagnosis and a course of action.

4. Explain the reason scanning for and reporting nuchal cord is controversial.

5. Discuss a cause of facial cleft.

IMAGE EVALUATION/PATHOLOGY

Review the images and answer the following questions.

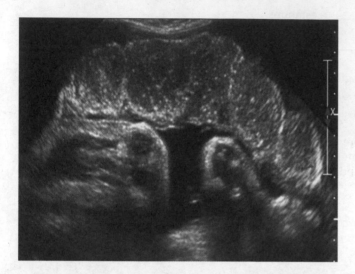

1. Describe the placenta.

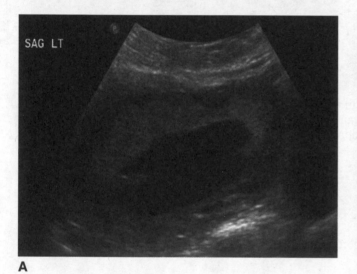

A

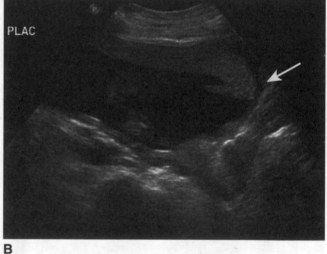

B

2. Identify the condition demonstrated in the images.

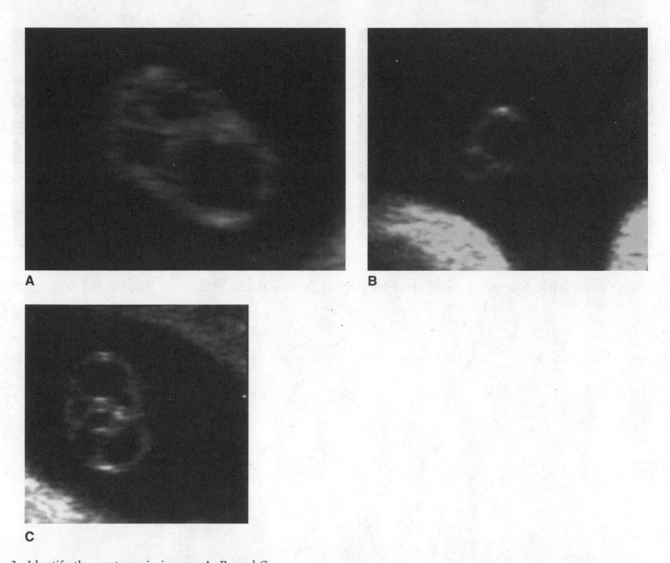

3. Identify the anatomy in images A, B, and C.

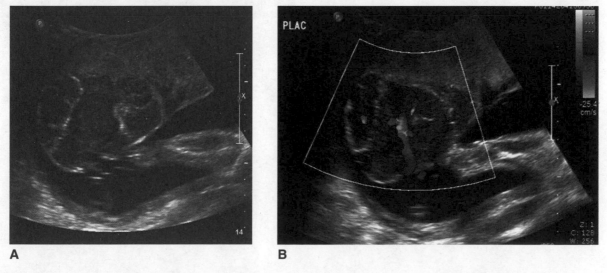

4. Image A reveals a large ovoid mass in 2D. Image B reveals the same mass with color Doppler sonography demonstrating vascularity within. Diagnose the anatomy.

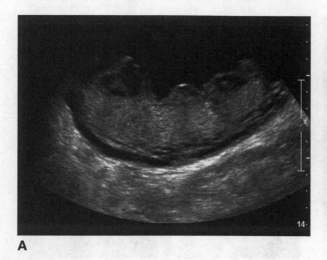
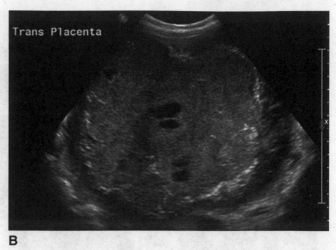

A   B

5. Diagnose the hypoechoic lesions noted within the placenta. Note: real-time sonography demonstrated swirling with the lesions.

CHAPTER 23

Sonographic Assessment of the Fetal Head

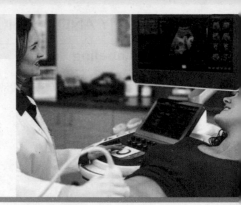

REVIEW OF GLOSSARY TERMS

Matching

Match the key terms with their definitions.

KEY TERMS

1. _____ anophthalmia

2. _____ brachycephaly

3. _____ cebocephaly

4. _____ colpocephaly

5. _____ dysgenesis

6. _____ dysmorphic

7. _____ dolichocephaly

8. _____ ectasia

9. _____ nares

10. _____ neuropore

11. _____ nomogram

12. _____ pathognomonic

13. _____ retrognathia

14. _____ rostral

15. _____ teratogen

16. _____ vermis

DEFINITIONS

a. Congenital brain anomaly resulting from a migrational defect of the occipital horns of the lateral ventricles leading to ventricular enlargement

b. Long narrow head

c. Graph

d. Dilatation or distension of a hollow structure

e. Posterior displacement of the maxilla and mandible

f. Congenital absence of one or both eyes

g. Either the rostral or caudal end of the neural tube

h. Toward the cephalic or head end

i. Congenital anomalies of the head owing to teratogens or development disruptions of the nervous system

j. Abnormally formed organs

k. Central portion of the cerebellum between the hemispheres

l. Short broad head owing to premature suture fusion

m. Nostrils

n. Disease characteristic

o. Malformation of an organ or structure

p. Substance that interferes with embryonic development

ANATOMY AND PHYSIOLOGY REVIEW

Image Labeling

Complete the labels in the images that follow.

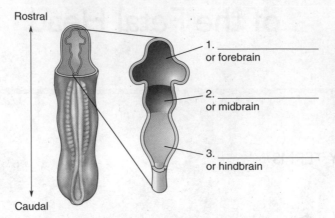

Three primary brain vesicles.

NORMAL VENTRICLES

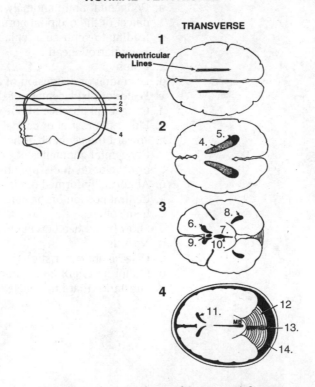

Drawing of ventricles and intracranial anatomy.

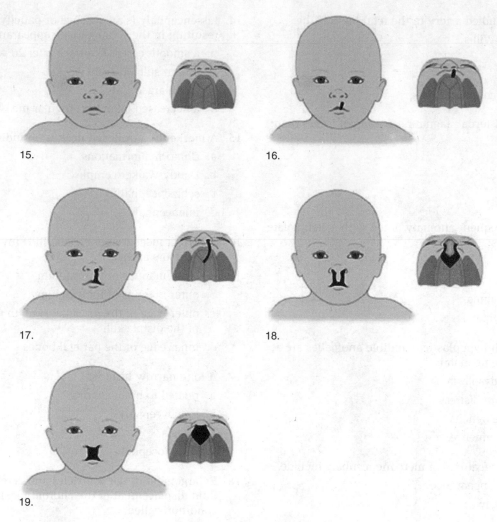

15.

16.

17.

18.

19.

Classification of common facial clefts.

CHAPTER REVIEW

Multiple Choice

Complete each question by circling the best answer.

1. The choroid plexus:
   a. invaginates into the ventricles
   b. is hyperechoic
   c. is positioned in the anterior ventricle
   d. initially takes up approximately 1/3 of the cerebral hemisphere

2. The metencephalon and myelencephalon are part of the:
   a. myelencephalon
   b. prosencephalon
   c. rhombencephalon
   d. mesencephalon

3. The corpus callosum, cerebellar vermis, sulci, gyri, migration of the germinal matrix, and myelination, develop after
   a. 12 weeks' gestation
   b. 15 weeks' gestation
   c. 18 weeks' gestation
   d. 20 weeks' gestation

4. BPD is measured at the level of the _____ and columns of the fornix.
   a. cisterna magna
   b. third ventricle
   c. thalami
   d. parietal sutures

5. What is the alternative measurement to the BPD?
   a. FL
   b. HL
   c. AC
   d. HC

6. The most studied artery in the fetal brain is the:
   a. circle of Willis
   b. MCA
   c. ICA
   d. anterior communicating

7. A normal cisterna magna measurement is less than:
   a. 4 mm
   b. 1 cm
   c. 8 mm
   d. 1.5 cm

8. The most frequent anomaly noted with a cleft palate or cleft lip is:
   a. clubfoot
   b. enlarged forehead
   c. anophthalmia
   d. retrognathia

9. Fetuses with hypoplastic mandible anomalies are at risk of acute neonatal:
   a. skeletal dysplasia
   b. respiratory distress
   c. cognitive deficits
   d. chin prominence

10. Sonographic features of meroanencephaly include:
    a. frog-like appearance
    b. polydactyly
    c. CP
    d. oligohydramnios

11. A fetal brain with no recognizable cerebral cortex and defined thalami and cerebellum is:
    a. holoprosencephaly
    b. CL
    c. hydranencephaly
    d. acrania

12. Agenesis of the corpus callosum reveals all except:
    a. wide high third ventricle
    b. laterally displaced ventricles
    c. absent cavum septi pellucidi
    d. hypertelorism

13. Dandy-Walker malformation consists of:
    a. hypertrophy of the third ventricle
    b. marked cystic dilation of the fourth ventricle
    c. marked cystic dilation of the lateral ventricles
    d. enlargement of the anterior horns

14. Lissencephaly is an absence or paucity of gyri resulting in the characteristic appearance of:
    a. a smooth cerebral surface after 20 weeks
    b. absent sulci after 20 weeks
    c. an enlarged CM
    d. a decreased lateral ventricular measurement

15. A markedly retroflexed neck is an indication of:
    a. Chiari malformations
    b. Dandy-Walker complex
    c. schizencephaly
    d. iniencephaly

16. A correct measurement of the BPD involves placing two cursors at the:
    a. inner margins of the cranium
    b. outer margins of the cranium
    c. outer edge of the proximal skull to the inner edge of the distal skull
    d. inner edge of the parietal bones

17. A long narrow head is:
    a. related to brain sparing
    b. brachycephaly
    c. ectasia
    d. dolichocephaly

18. Enlargement of the ventricles and cerebrospinal fluid displacement of the choroid plexus results in a condition called:
    a. dangling choroid plexus
    b. teardrop ventricle
    c. cebocephalic
    d. cephalic pole

19. Bleeding anywhere in the fetal cranium is known as all except:
    a. intraparenchymal hemorrhage
    b. subdural hematoma
    c. germinal matrix hemorrhage
    d. petechial hemorrhage

20. A measurement of the lateral ventricular atrium should not exceed:
    a. 1 cm
    b. 1 mm
    c. 8 mm
    d. 2 cm

Fill-in-the-Blank

1. The forebrain is also known as the _____.

2. Many brain structures develop between week _____, resulting in this time frame being identified as the critical period of brain development.

3. The great cerebral vein is also called _____.

4. The third ventricle is positioned between the _____ and the frontal horns of the lateral ventricles.

5. A microcephalic fetus may demonstrate _____ ventricles.

6. The best angle of insonation to obtain peak velocity of the MCA is less than _____ degrees.

7. A decreased interorbital distance is _____.

8. Between _____ weeks of gestation, the transverse cerebellar diameter measured in millimeters correlates 1:1 with the gestational age.

9. Holoprosencephaly is divided into _____, _____, and _____ varieties, defined by the degree of separation of the cerebral hemispheres.

10. _____ is a cerebral developmental disorder that involves disordered neuronal migration.

11. Protrusions of the meninges and frequently of brain substance through a defect in the cranium is _____.

12. The term for small head is _____.

13. To obtain the MCA peak velocity, image the fetal head in a _____ plane.

14. The presence of a single median bony orbit with a fleshy proboscis above it is _____.

15. Arnold-Chiari malformations often have accompanying _____.

16. The BPD maintains its closest correlation with gestational age in the _____ and _____ trimesters.

17. _____ is an abnormal increase in the volume of the cerebral ventricles.

18. A sonolucent area in the choroid plexus is known as _____.

19. Macrocephaly is defined as a head circumference _____ standard deviations _____ the mean for gestational age and sex.

20. The tongue extending beyond the teeth or alveolar ridge is _____.

Short Answer

1. Explain microcephaly.

2. What are cranial structure alternative methods of determining the age of a fetus other than BPD, HC, AC, and FL?

3. Discuss cephalocele and encephalocele and cranial meningocele.

IMAGE EVALUATION/PATHOLOGY

Review the images and answer the following questions.

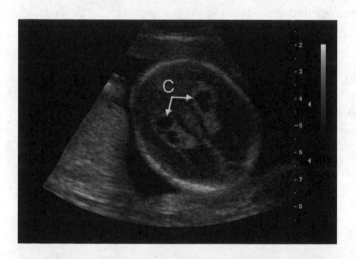

1. Name the structure the arrows are directed toward.

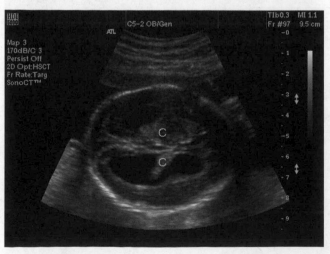

2. Explain the image and offer a diagnosis.

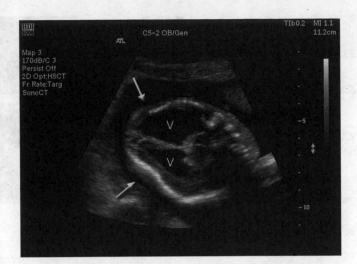

3. State the name of this cranial anomaly.

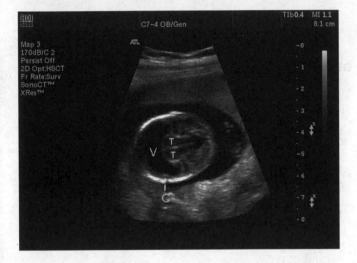

4. Offer a diagnosis.

CHAPTER 24

Sonographic Assessment of the Fetal Neck and Spine

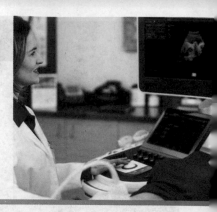

REVIEW OF GLOSSARY TERMS

Matching

Match the key terms with their definitions.

KEY TERMS

1. _____ neuropore

2. _____ pluripotent

3. _____ dysgenesis

4. _____ omphalocele

5. _____ gastroschisis

6. _____ lipoma

7. _____ lymphangiectasia

8. _____ myeloschisis

9. _____ myelomeningocele

10. _____ meningocele

DEFINITIONS

a. Abnormally formed organs
b. Combination of nonimmune fetal hydrops and a cystic hygroma
c. Herniation of abdominal contents without a covering into the amniotic fluid
d. Spinal defect where the meninges protrude
e. Protrusion of a sac from a spinal defect that contains spinal cord and meninges
f. Incomplete fusion of the neural tube resulting in a cleft spinal cord
g. Herniation of the abdominal contents with a membranous cover
h. Tumor composed of fat
i. Either the rostral or caudal end of the neural tube
j. Ability of embryonic cells to differentiate into any type of cell

ANATOMY AND PHYSIOLOGY REVIEW

Image Labeling

Complete the labels in the images that follow.

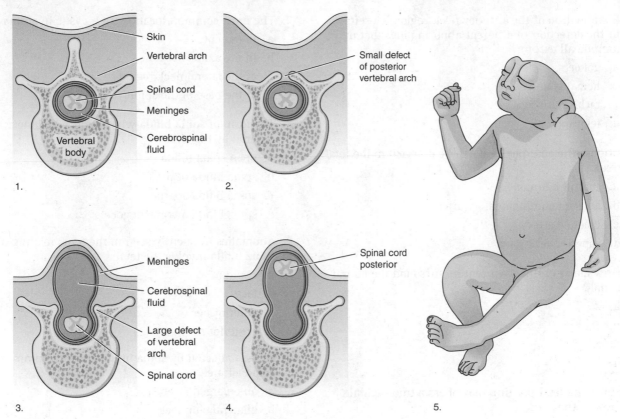

1.

2.

3.

4.

5.

Neural tube defects

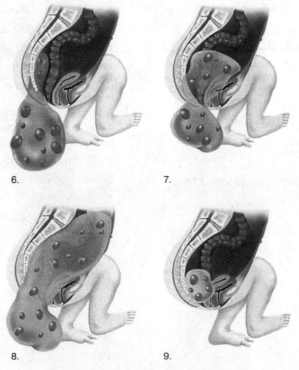

6.

7.

8.

9.

Sacrococcygeal teratomas

CHAPTER REVIEW

Multiple Choice

Complete each question by circling the best answer.

1. Examination of the anterior neck region is useful in the detection of different abnormalities that may include all except:
   a. goiter
   b. hemangioma
   c. rachischisis
   d. teratoma

2. Choose the anatomy that can be detected in the fetal neck.
   a. carotid bifurcation
   b. anterior communicating artery
   c. brachial artery
   d. superior vena cava

3. How many ossification centers surround the neural canal?
   a. 2
   b. 3
   c. 5
   d. 7

4. Select the fetal position that offers a true sagittal view of the spine.
   a. transverse
   b. oblique
   c. cephalic
   d. prone

5. Determination of spinal normalcy is through identification of all except:
   a. an intact neural canal
   b. divergence of the posterior ossification elements
   c. a normal location and shape of spinal ossification centers
   d. an intact dorsal skin contour

6. Screening for neural tube defects is performed by all except:
   a. hCG
   b. sonography
   c. MSAFP
   d. biochemical testing

7. The most common location for a cystic hygroma is:
   a. in the chest
   b. in the axillary region
   c. at the lateral neck region
   d. at the base of the spine

8. The form of spina bifida where split vertebrae are covered by the skin is:
   a. open spina bifida
   b. spina bifida occulta
   c. spina bifida aperta
   d. spina bifida myomeningocele

9. Anomalies frequently seen in the fetus relating to spina bifida involve the fetal:
   a. cranium
   b. face
   c. anterior neck
   d. posterior neck

10. Fetuses affected by spina bifida aperta commonly demonstrate:
    a. an enlarged forehead
    b. bilateral club feet
    c. polydactyly
    d. clenched hands

11. Scoliosis is an abnormal:
    a. anterior angulation of the spine
    b. posterior angulation of the spine
    c. lateral curvature of the spine
    d. thoracic defect of the spine

12. A term that refers to a heterogeneous group of congenital anomalies affecting the distal spine and cord, the hindgut, the urogenital system, and the lower limbs is:
    a. disruption canalization
    b. lumbar/sacral absence
    c. sirenomelia
    d. caudal regression syndrome

13. A sacrococcygeal teratoma most commonly images as a protrusion:
    a. at the umbilical cord insertion
    b. at the thoracic region
    c. at the lumbar region
    d. between the anus and the coccyx

14. The earliest visible indication of caudal regression syndrome is:
    a. a short crown–rump length and abnormal yolk sac
    b. renal anomalies
    c. gastrointestinal anomalies
    d. lack of lower extremity movement during an ultrasound examination

15. Cystic hygromas are the result of _____ obstruction, usually occurring in the head or neck region.
    a. trachea
    b. tumor
    c. carotid vessel
    d. lymph vessel

Fill-in-the-Blank

1. The normal fetal spine has _____ ossification centers: the centrum, right, and left neural processes.

2. The fetal spine images with brightly echogenic ossification centers in the transverse plane by the _____ week of gestation.

3. Three types of scanning planes help with the evaluation of spinal integrity: _____, _____, and _____.

4. AFP is elevated in NTD, other open fetal defects, such as _____ and _____, as well as skin disorders that increase the diffusion of AFP through fetal skin.

5. Cystic hygromas appear as either single or _____ fluid-filled cavities and are usually located on the _____ neck.

6. The two types of spina bifida lesions are _____ and _____. The most common form of the process is _____ spina bifida.

7. The location and severity of spina bifida have the greatest chance of detection on _____ views.

8. Fusion of the fetal legs is known as the _____ syndrome, also known as _____.

9. The most common location of a neural tube teratoma is the _____ end.

10. Sagittal and coronal images of _____ and spinal anatomy assist in detecting spinal normalcy or assist in locating anomalous deviations.

Short Answer

1. A concerned patient has questions about the MSAFP screening. Explain the test and reasons for performing it, and what can be determined by the results.

2. Two clearly defined legs are not seen in a 21-week fetus during a level I screening ultrasound. Offer a diagnosis and differential diagnosis.

IMAGE EVALUATION/PATHOLOGY

Review the images and answer the following questions.

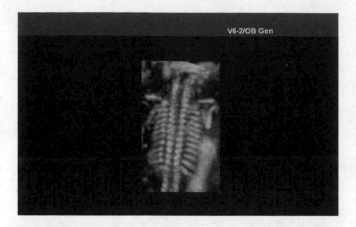

1. Identify the anatomy displayed. Is it normal or abnormal? State the type of imaging that produced the image.

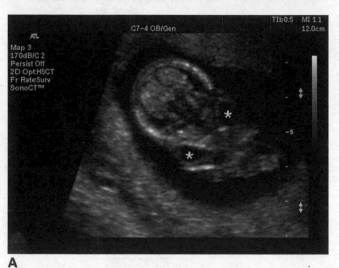

A

B

2. What is the diagnosis? Note asterisks.

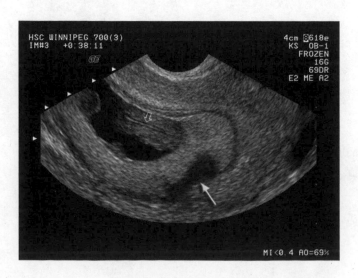

3. Describe the anatomy depicted by the open arrow. Is it normal? Note: This is an 8-week fetus.

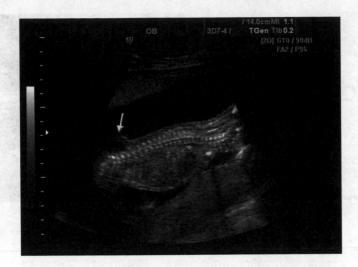

4. Identify anatomy and the anomaly in the image (see arrow).

CHAPTER 25

Fetal Echocardiography

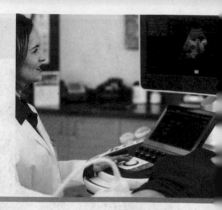

REVIEW OF GLOSSARY TERMS

Matching

Match the key terms with their definitions.

KEY TERMS

1. _____ double-outlet right ventricle (DORV)

2. _____ rhabdomyoma

3. _____ akinetic

4. _____ dextrocardia

5. _____ right ventricular hypoplasia (hypoplastic right heart)

6. _____ ventricular septal defect (VSD)

7. _____ ductus venosus

8. _____ premature atrial contractions (PACs)

9. _____ arrhythmia

10. _____ truncus arteriosus

11. _____ dyskinetic

12. _____ atrial septal defect (ASD)

13. _____ tricuspid atresia

14. _____ septum primum

15. _____ Ebstein anomaly

16. _____ papillary muscles

17. _____ coarctation of the aorta

DEFINITIONS

a. Abnormal heart rate

b. Without motion

c. Partial: Primum type ASD in the lower portion of the atrial septum without a ventricular defect component; complete: a heart with both primum type ASD and inlet type VSD and a single, common atrioventricular valve

d. Abnormal opening between the right and left atrium

e. Slow heart rate

f. Valves located between the atrium and ventricles (tricuspid and mitral valves)

g. Apex of the heart points to the right

h. Narrowing of the aorta, either discreet or long segment

i. Venous connection from the umbilical vein inserting into the inferior vena cava

j. Both great arteries arise from the morphologic right ventricle, with a VSD. There may be pulmonary stenosis and/or other lesions present.

k. Right heart abnormality with apical displacement of the tricuspid valve resulting in varying degrees of right atrial enlargement or diminished RV size and function, tricuspid regurgitation, and possible pulmonary stenosis or atresia

l. Impaired or abnormal movement

m. Calculation of the heart to chest size resulting in a ratio

n. Normal opening in the atrial septum allowing for blood flow from the right to left atrium during fetal life

o. Subset of cells found in the developing heart tube that will give rise to the heart's atrioventricular valves and septae; critical to the proper formation of a four-chambered heart

18. _____ transposition of the great arteries (TGA)

19. _____ endocardial cushion

20. _____ hydrops, nonimmune

21. _____ bradyarrhythmia

22. _____ atrioventricular septal defects (AVSD, endocardial cushion defect)

23. _____ Tetralogy of Fallot

24. _____ foramen ovale

25. _____ atrioventricular valves (AVs)

26. _____ hypoplastic left heart syndrome (HLHS)

27. _____ supraventricular tachycardia (SVT)

28. _____ heart/thorax ratio (CTR)

p. Underdevelopment of the left heart, in particular, the mitral valve, the left ventricle, and aorta; stenosis or atresia of the aortic and/or mitral valves

q. Accumulation of fluid in the chest and abdomen because of heart failure

r. Irregular extra contraction of the atria; may be conducted or blocked in relation to the ventricles

s. Muscular projections into the ventricles that anchor the chordae tendineae of the AV valves

t. Most common benign fetal cardiac tumor. Associated with the genetic disorder tuberous sclerosis complex

u. Single semilunar (truncal) valve providing both pulmonary artery and aortic arch flow; VSD

v. A deficiency in the ventricular septum creating a communication and blood flow between the ventricles

w. Cardiac malformation where the aorta arises from the morphologic right ventricle and the pulmonary artery arises from the morphologic left ventricle

x. Congenital absence/closure of the tricuspid valve

y. Fast sustained heartbeat/arrhythmia. Not ventricular in origin; may originate from the atria, AV node, sinoatrial node, or as a result of an additional electrical bypass tract

z. Cardiac malformation with a VSD, anterior malaligned conal septum, varying degrees of pulmonary stenosis, overriding aorta

aa. First section/side of the interatrial septum to form in the embryo

bb. Underdevelopment of the right ventricle and the tricuspid valve

ANATOMY AND PHYSIOLOGY REVIEW

Image Labeling

Complete the labels in the images that follow.

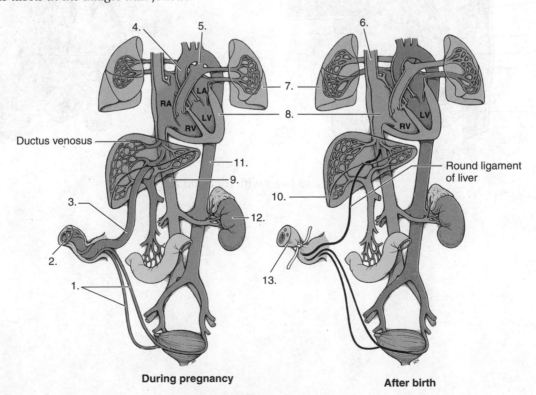

During pregnancy

After birth

Fetal and newborn circulation

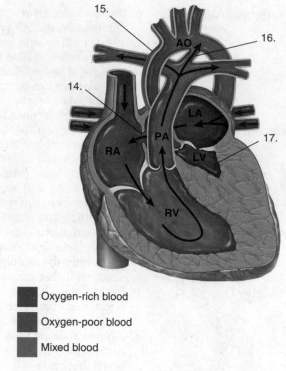

Oxygen-rich blood

Oxygen-poor blood

Mixed blood

Hypoplastic left heart syndrome

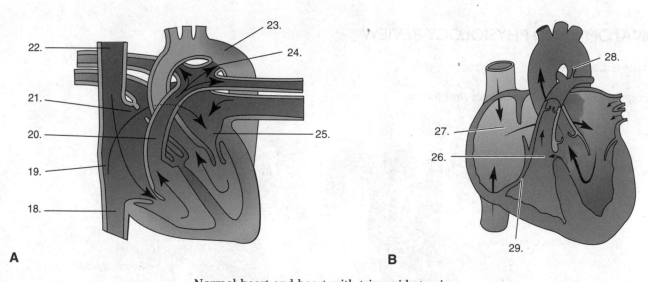

A

B

Normal heart and heart with tricuspid atresia

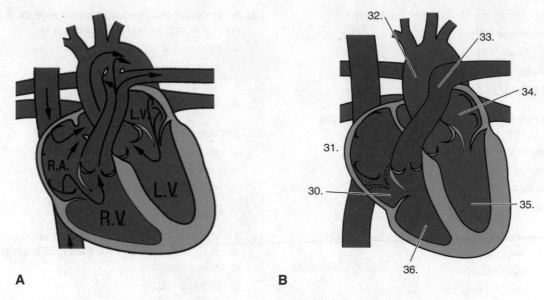

Normal heart and heart with Ebstein anomaly

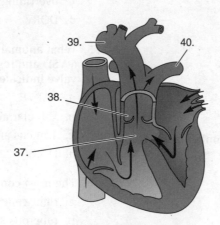

Persistent truncus arteriosus

CHAPTER REVIEW

Multiple Choice

Complete each question by circling the best answer.

1. The embryonic heart is completely formed at the:
   a. beginning of the seventh week
   b. beginning of the eighth week
   c. end of the seventh week
   d. end of the eighth week

2. Fetal blood circulates within the embryo at:
   a. 2 weeks postconception
   b. 6 weeks gestational age
   c. 3 weeks postconception
   d. 4 weeks gestational age

3. Fetal oxygenated blood circulation from the placenta enters the fetus through the:
   a. umbilical vein to the hepatic circulation and left portal vein
   b. umbilical vein to the ductus arteriosus and right atrium
   c. umbilical artery to the ductus venosus and left portal vein
   d. umbilical artery to the left portal vein and IVC

4. Fetal blood from the IVC enters the heart:
   a. left ventricle (LV)
   b. right ventricle (RV)
   c. left atrium (LV)
   d. right atrium (RA)

5. In the fetus, left atrial blood passes through the _____ into the left ventricle.
   a. tricuspid valve
   b. pulmonary valve
   c. semilunar valve
   d. mitral valve

6. The greatest concentration of oxygenated fetal blood travels to the:
   a. abdominal organs
   b. retroperitoneal organs
   c. cranium
   d. distal extremities

7. A normal heart orientation is:
   a. levocardia
   b. dextrocardia
   c. mesocardia
   d. dextroposition

8. In the normal fetal heart, which chamber is located closest to the fetal spine?
   a. Left atrium (LA)
   b. Right atrium (RA)
   c. Left ventricle (RV)
   d. Right ventricle (RA)

9. Fetal tachyarrhythmias are heart rates:
   a. more than 180 beats per minute
   b. less than 100 beats per minute
   c. best assessed using Doppler
   d. usually clinically insignificant

10. Digoxin, sotalol, and flecainide are most often selected for fetal treatment of:
    a. complete heart block
    b. SVT
    c. PAC
    d. VSD

11. A defect of the inlet, outlet, trabecular, or apical portion of the fetal septum involves the:
    a. muscular septum
    b. heart apex
    c. moderator band
    d. endocardial cushion

12. A syndrome that includes aortic atresia, a small left ventricle, and mitral valve atresia is:
    a. pulmonary atresia
    b. tricuspid atresia
    c. HLHS
    d. aortic coarctation

13. Tetralogy of Fallot includes all except:
    a. perimembranous VSD
    b. right atrial hypertrophy
    c. pulmonic stenosis
    d. pulmonary artery hypoplasia

14. An abnormally large right atrium and abnormally small right ventricle with tricuspid regurgitation is an indication of:
    a. Ebstein anomaly
    b. TGA
    c. overriding aorta
    d. DORV

15. What anomaly describes a single vessel overriding a VSD and regurgitant flow, and thickened stenotic valve indicate?
    a. TAPVR
    b. Valvular atresia
    c. Truncus arteriosus
    d. DORV

16. The most common cardiac tumor is:
    a. right ventricular teratoma
    b. tuberous sclerosis
    c. DiGeorge syndrome
    d. rhabdomyoma

17. DORV involves:
    a. severe ASD
    b. a conotruncal defect with the aorta and pulmonary artery failing to divide
    c. more than 50% of both the aortic root and PA arise from the morphologic RV
    d. premature closure of the foramen ovale

18. Ostium primum and ostium secundum defects involve the:
    a. ventricular septum
    b. atrial septum
    c. moderator septum
    d. IVC

19. The pulmonary valve receives blood from the:
    a. right atrium
    b. left atrium
    c. right ventricle
    d. left ventricle

20. Current ultrasound resolution limits of _____ mm may prevent the identification of small VSDs.
    a. 1 to 2
    b. 2 to 3
    c. 3 to 4
    d. 4 to 5

Fill-in-the-Blank

1. Blood begins to circulate in the embryo at _____ weeks postconception, which is _____ weeks gestational age.

2. The fetal heart should consume most of the _____ side of the chest and lays with a normal angle of _____ degrees to the _____ of midline, plus or minus 20 degrees. The normal position of the heart is termed _____.

3. A right-sided heart with the apex pointing left is called _____. A heart positioned in the right chest with the apex pointing right is labeled _____. A midline heart is termed _____.

4. The standard first view in an echocardiogram is the _____ view.

5. The subcostal fetal heart view is used for the _____ view, _____ view of the ventricles, and Doppler interrogation of the _____.

6. A long axis view of the _____ artery demonstrates the RVOT. A long axis view of the _____ demonstrates the LVOT.

7. The brachiocephalic, left common carotid, and left subclavian artery arise from the _____ arch, which has a _____ shape or appearance.

8. A fetal sustained heart rate of 100 bpm or less is called _____.

9. The most frequent cardiac malformation is _____, occurring in about 30% of live births.

10. The three bypasses of the fetal heart that close at parturition are _____, _____, and _____.

11. The 3D imaging mode used specifically for fetal cardiac imaging is _____.

12. Tricuspid atresia results in _____ hypoplasia. It appears as a _____, _____ valve.

13. Narrowing of the aorta along the arch is _____ and results in possible _____ descending aortic flow distal to ductus arteriosus entrance.

14. Complete TGA is _____ and _____ concordant connection; aorta originating from the _____; pulmonary artery originating from the _____.

15. Endocardial cushion defect is also known as _____.

16. The _____ view of the fetal heart is often used for the diagnosis of VSD.

17. Tubular structures called _____ are the first development of the fetal heart.

18. Chamber dilation proximal to an atretic valve is known as _____.

19. The _____ is the most common solid, benign cardiac mass seen in the fetus.

20. The correct flow direction through the foramen ovale is _____ to _____.

21. A structure in the right ventricle, the _____, should differentiate the right ventricle from the left ventricle.

22. The structure that separates the right and left ventricular chambers is the _____.

23. The foraminal flap should be seen opening into the _____ atrium.

24. Tetralogy of Fallot is the result of six defects: a _____, _____, _____, _____, _____, and _____.

25. _____ is a condition in which the aortic root and pulmonary artery arise from the right ventricle.

26. Failure of the embryonic truncus to separate into the aorta and pulmonary artery is known as _____.

Short Answer

1. In the case of suspected arrhythmia, where on the fetal heart should M-mode tracings be performed?

2. Describe the most diagnostic views for diagnosing Ebstein anomaly.

3. Name the two cardiac malformations displayed by parallel great vessels?

4. What is fluid in the fetal chest most often called and caused by?

5. What single view best demonstrates truncus arteriosus?

IMAGE EVALUATION/PATHOLOGY

Review the images and answer the following questions.

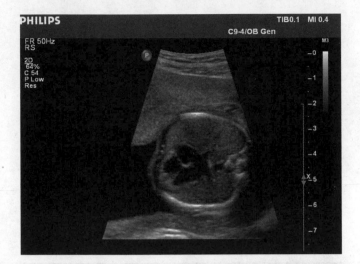

1. Diagnose the single image.

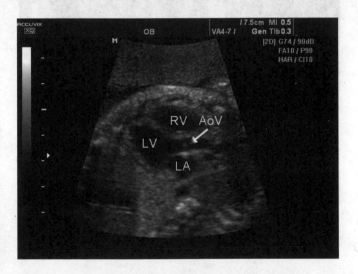

2. Describe the view and state the name of the structure exiting the left ventricle. Explain the labels LV, RV, LA, and AoV.

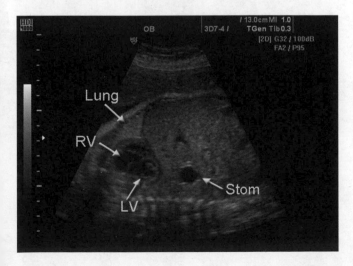

3. Name the view of the ventricles. Name the structure seen in the left ventricle that the arrow points toward.

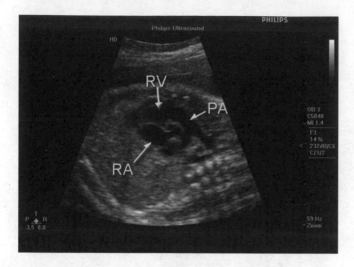

4. What valve is seen between the RV and RA?

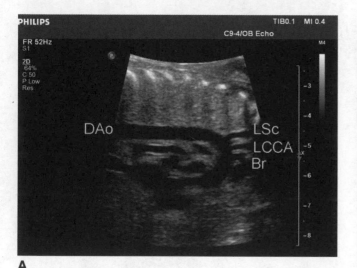

A

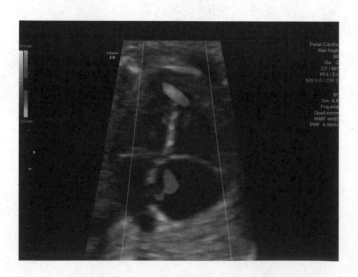

B

5. A. Describe the fetal position. B. Name the vessels seen at the aortic arch.

6. Offer a diagnosis. Pay close attention to the apical septum.

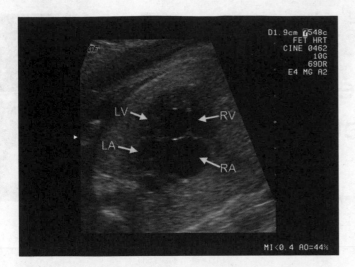

7. Diagnose the image.

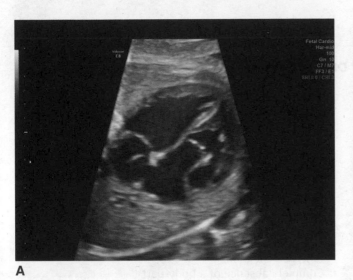

A

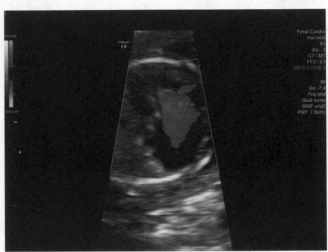

B

8. Explain the 2D image and offer a diagnosis.

CHAPTER 26

Sonographic Assessment of the Fetal Chest

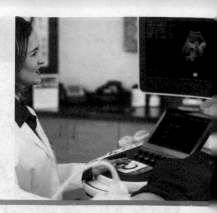

REVIEW OF GLOSSARY TERMS

Matching

Match the key terms with their definitions.

KEY TERMS

1. _____ hypoplasia
2. _____ aplasia
3. _____ 4D imaging
4. _____ VOCAL
5. _____ bronchogenic cyst
6. _____ anasarca
7. _____ cardiomegaly
8. _____ pulmonary sequestration
9. _____ 3D imaging
10. _____ chorioamnionitis
11. _____ congenital diaphragmatic hernia (CDH)
12. _____ congenital multicystic adenomatoid malformation (CCAM)
13. _____ hemangioma
14. _____ Potter sequence
15. _____ mediastinum chest
16. _____ osteogenesis imperfecta
17. _____ look direction
18. _____ hypointense

DEFINITIONS

a. Adds motion to static 3D imaging, allowing for real-time 3D imaging of anatomy in motion
b. Semi-automated process to calculate volume using a 3D data set
c. Area lying between the lungs, which contains the heart, aorta, esophagus, trachea, and thymus
d. Accumulation of fluid in the fetal tissues, peritoneum, and pleural cavities owing to either immune or non-immune factors
e. Areas of high intensity or increased brightness on the magnetic resonance imaging (MRI) image; equivalent to hyperechogenic
f. Complete absence of a body part
g. Direction you are looking at a patient or structure (i.e., anterior to posterior)
h. Half-Fourier acquisition single-shot turbo spine-echo; a fast spin method to obtain the MRI data set
i. Underdevelopment or incomplete development of a body part
j. Generalized edema in the subcutaneous tissue
k. Birth defect of the diaphragm that allows the abdominal contents to enter the chest
l. Areas of low intensity or increased brightness on the MRI image; equivalent to hypoechogenic
m. Solitary cyst within the lung
n. Genetic disorder causing extremely fragile bones
o. Enlarged heart
p. Noncommunicating lung tissue that lacks pulmonary blood supply
q. Inflammation of the fetal membranes (amnion/chorion) owing to infection
r. Replacement of normal lung by nonfunctioning cystic lung tissue

19. _____ IUGR

20. _____ HASTE

21. _____ pulmonary hypoplasia

22. _____ hydrops

23. _____ hyperintense

s. Group of findings, also called Potter syndrome or oligohydramnios sequence, includes renal conditions such as agenesis, obstructive processes, and acquired or inherited cystic disease
t. Benign mass made up of blood vessels
u. Incomplete development of the lung tissue
v. Fetal weight below 10th percentile for gestational age
w. From a volume data set, static 3D images can display height, width, and depth of anatomy (three dimensions) from any orthogonal plane

CHAPTER REVIEW

Multiple Choice

Complete each question by circling the best answer.

1. The fetal chest should be evaluated for all except:
   a. L 1-5
   b. heart
   c. diaphragm
   d. bony symmetry

2. Routine observation of fetal breathing movements in the _____ trimester(s) should be included in the fetal examination.
   a. first and second
   b. first
   c. second and third
   d. third

3. The thoracic inlet is at the:
   a. level of the mouth
   b. base of the neck, level of clavicles
   c. base of the lungs
   d. level of C1

4. The fetal heart lies with the apex oriented toward the:
   a. liver
   b. stomach
   c. spleen
   d. gallbladder

5. A break in the skin surface directly over the spine is associated with:
   a. nonossified spinous processes
   b. convergence of the paired posterior ossified elements
   c. deleted spinous processes
   d. myelomeningocele

6. Thoracic chest measurements (outer edge to outer edge) are obtained from a true transverse view at the level of the:
   a. fetal heart
   b. three-vessel view
   c. cardiac apex
   d. widest portion of the lung

7. If the fetal heart (in transverse view) occupies more the 1/3 of the thorax, _____ should be considered:
   a. pulmonary hypoplasia
   b. cardiac hypoplasia
   c. pulmonary hyperplasia
   d. cardiac hyperplasia

8. Fetal lung development begins in what week?
   a. Third
   b. Fourth
   c. Sixth
   d. Eighth

9. Respiration becomes possible during the _____ week because of the development of terminal saccules.
   a. 20th
   b. 24th
   c. 26th
   d. 28th

10. Fetal lung volume can be estimated by all except:
    a. MRI
    b. VOCAL
    c. 3D data set
    d. 2D coronal

11. Successfully locating the oropharynx and laryngeal pharynx is accomplished with a:
    a. longitudinal view through the upper neck and an empty pharynx
    b. transverse view through the upper neck and an empty pharynx
    c. longitudinal view through the upper neck and a fluid-filled pharynx
    d. transverse view through the upper neck and a fluid-filled pharynx

12. Lung masses include all except:
    a. CCAM
    b. aortic aneurysm
    c. teratoma
    d. pulmonary atresia

13. CCAM typically appears as all except:
    a. a bilateral large predominantly cystic mass of the lower lobes
    b. a unilateral pulmonary mass with one or more large cysts
    c. an echogenic mass containing small cysts
    d. a homogeneous echogenic mass

14. The presence of abnormal and excessive skin or soft tissue in the nuchal area is a well-known and common clinical finding in many newborns with Trisomy 21 and is suspect if the nuchal fold measures:
    a. 2 mm or greater in 8 to 11 weeks
    b. 2 mm or greater in 11 to 13 weeks
    c. 4 mm or greater in 19 to 24 weeks
    d. 6 mm or greater in 19 to 24 weeks

15. Fetal posterolateral neck thickening may be caused by all except:
    a. absent clavicles
    b. failure of the lymphatic channels to communicate
    c. nuchal skin thickening
    d. Turner syndrome

16. The most accurate term for a collection of lymph within the chest is referred to as:
    a. hydrothorax
    b. chylothorax
    c. pleural effusion
    d. milky effusion

17. Nonimmune fetal hydrops is related to:
    a. erythroblastosis fetalis
    b. severe anemia
    c. severe fetal disease
    d. Rh incompatibility

18. The AC measurement in a fetus with CDH:
    a. is smaller than normal
    b. is larger than normal
    c. is normal
    d. displays ascites

Fill-in-the-Blank

1. The correct area to obtain thoracic measurements is from a true transverse view just above the _____ at the level of the fetal _____.

2. _____ is the gold standard for indication of fetal lung maturity.

3. The _____ is located at the level of the great vessel of the heart, anterior to the aorta and pulmonary artery.

4. The typical scapula has a sonographic appearance of a _____ or _____ shape, depending on the angle of insonation.

5. The muscles of the chest wall are _____ echoic and thin.

6. The lungs are separated from these abdominal organs by the _____.

7. _____ remains the gold standard in accessing lung maturity.

8. The fetal diaphragm is seen as a thin, hypoechoic, dome-shaped muscular band separating the _____ cavities from echogenic _____ tissue.

9. Pleural effusions are an accumulation of _____ fluid in the fetal lungs.

10. To differentiate pulmonary sequestration from CCAM, use color Doppler to trace the origin of _____ _____.

11. Both fetal edema and cystic hygroma have an increased connection with _____ abnormalities.

12. Cystic hygromas are thought to be a result of a failure in the development of normal _____ venous communication.

13. Compression on the esophagus by a mass could lead to _____ because of GI tract obstruction.

14. Mass compression on the vena cava may compromise blood return to the fetal heart and lead to the development of _____.

15. The thymus is located at the level of the great vessel of the heart, _____ to the aorta and pulmonary artery.

16. The _____ enlarges with immune fetal hydrops and infections.

17. _____ is the most frequently found mass within the fetal chest.

18. Imaging the diaphragm can help differentiate cystic intrathoracic masses of pulmonary origin from those that are of _____ origin.

Short Answer

1. Describe the appearance of a normal diaphragm.

2. How is CCAM viewed differently from pulmonary sequestration using ultrasound? Will MRI as a complementary imaging modality be helpful to differentiate the two processes?

3. Explain immune fetal hydrops and compare it with nonimmune fetal hydrops.

IMAGE EVALUATION/PATHOLOGY

Review the images and answer the following questions.

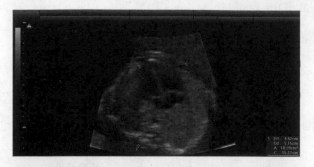

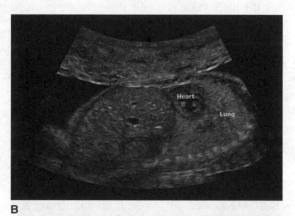

1. Name the view. Explain the reason a dotted circular line is seen.

2. What are the arrows pointing at?

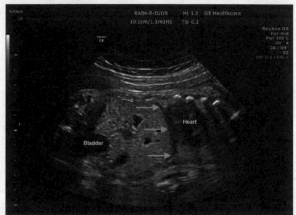

A

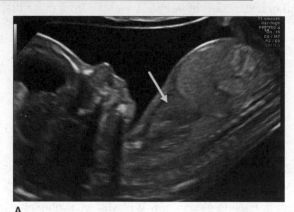

B

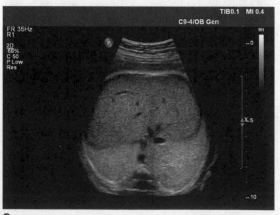

C

3. Name the structure seen in all three images. Image A shows an arrow directed toward it.

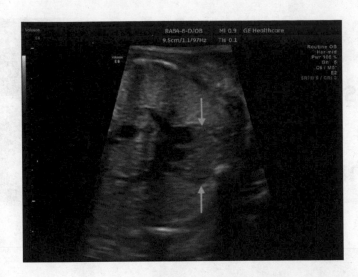

4. Name the structures at the arrow ends. Describe the appearance of it compared to the adjacent anatomy.

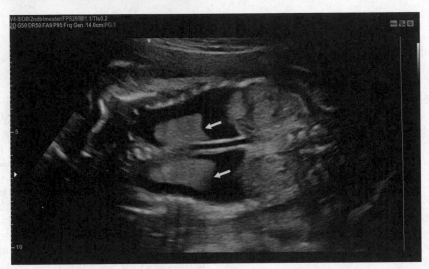

5. Diagnose the image.

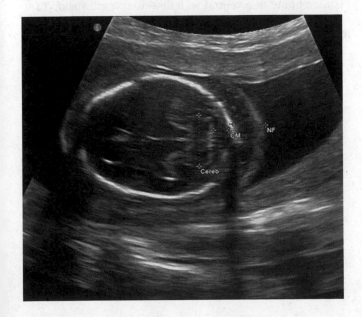

6. Explain the image. Offer a diagnosis.

CHAPTER 27

Sonographic Assessment of the Fetal Abdomen (Includes Abdominal Wall)

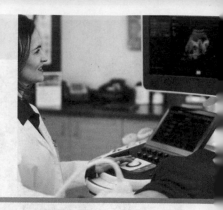

REVIEW OF GLOSSARY TERMS

Matching

Match the key terms with their definitions.

KEY TERMS

1. _____ biliary atresia

2. _____ upper GI

3. _____ trisomy

4. _____ situs inversus

5. _____ parvovirus infection

6. _____ omphalocele

7. _____ midgut volvulus

8. _____ myelomeningocele (spina bifida)

9. _____ meconium ileus

10. _____ isointense

11. _____ hypointense

12. _____ hyperintense

13. _____ ascites

14. _____ Hirschsprung disease

15. _____ hematopoiesis

16. _____ HASTE

17. _____ gastroschisis

18. _____ duodenal atresia

DEFINITIONS

a. Half-Fourier acquisition single-shot turbo spine-echo; a fast spin method to obtain the MRI data set

b. Congenital blockage or absence of the bile duct

c. Bowel obstructed owing to bowel twisting

d. Disorder where the spinal cord does not close before birth

e. Genetic abnormality where there is the presence of three copies of a particular chromosome

f. Areas of similar intensity or increased brightness on the MRI image; equivalent to isoechoic

g. Accumulation of fluid in the abdominal cavity

h. Reversal of normal organ position

i. Congenital lack of nerves in the colon resulting in fecal impaction and a megacolon

j. Congenital absence or closing of the duodenal lumen

k. Membrane-covered ventral wall defect containing abdominal contents involving the umbilical cord

l. Membrane-free ventral wall defect with protrusion of abdominal contents lateral to the umbilical cord

m. Formation of blood cells

n. Radiographic study using barium sulfate as a contrast agent to outline and fill the gastrointestinal tract

o. Areas of low intensity or decreased brightness on the MRI image; equivalent to hypoechogenic

p. Bowel obstructed by mucus

q. Congenital disorder caused by transplacental transmission of the parvovirus to the fetus, characterized by hydrops, ascites, ventriculomegaly, and other findings

r. Areas of high intensity or increased brightness on the magnetic resonance imaging (MRI) image; equivalent to hyperechogenic

ANATOMY AND PHYSIOLOGY REVIEW

Image Labeling

Complete the labels in the images that follow.

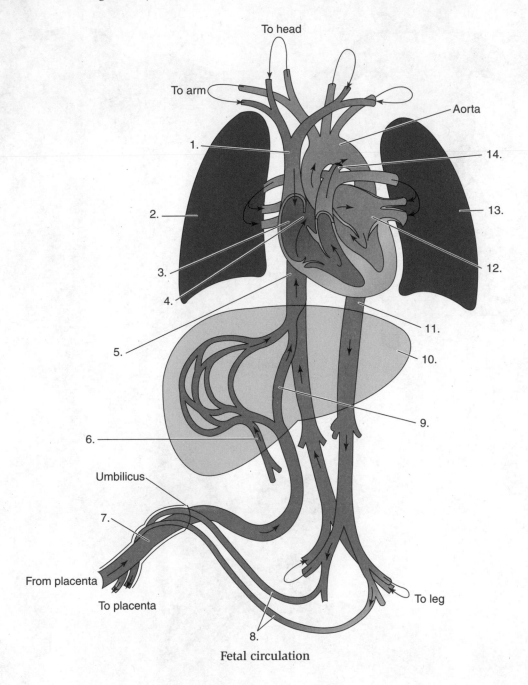

Fetal circulation

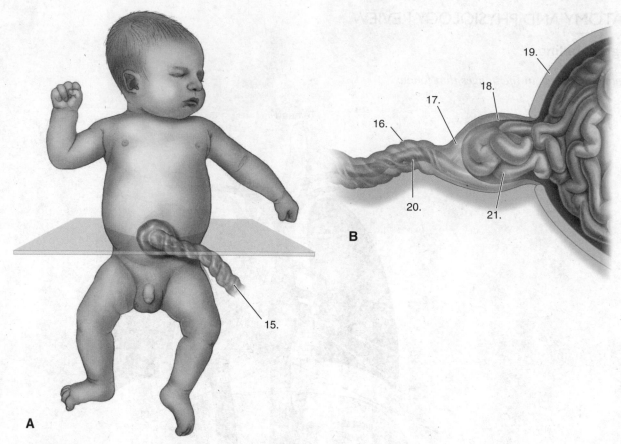

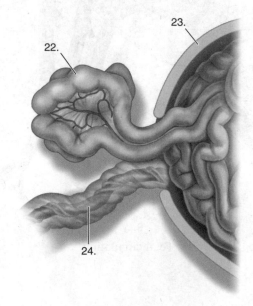

Omphalocele

Gastroschisis

CHAPTER REVIEW

Multiple Choice

Complete each question by circling the best answer.

1. The fetal organ that is usually not seen well in the second trimester is the:
   a. liver
   b. gallbladder
   c. pancreas
   d. kidney(s)

2. Left parasagittal views of the fetal abdomen demonstrate the:
   a. stomach and left kidney
   b. liver and right kidney
   c. umbilical entry
   d. diaphragm

3. The umbilical vein can be followed in a sagittal view from the anterior abdominal wall into the:
   a. main portal vein
   b. inferior vena cava
   c. ductus venosus
   d. liver's left portal vein

4. The allantois is:
   a. involved in early placental maturation
   b. involved in early blood production
   c. involved in the production of Wharton jelly
   d. a permanent structure

5. After birth, the ductus venosus closes and becomes the:
   a. fissure of ductus
   b. ligamentum venosum
   c. foramen ovale
   d. ligament of Treitz

6. Fetuses of diabetic mothers often display:
   a. increased abdominal circumference
   b. decreased abdominal circumference
   c. increased cranial circumference
   d. decreased cranial circumference

7. A correct AC measure includes the:
   a. fetal lungs
   b. ribs/spine
   c. soft tissue surrounding the ribs/spine
   d. kidneys

8. The spleen is part of the:
   a. digestive system
   b. neurologic system
   c. respiratory system
   d. lymphatic system

9. In a fetus, the spleen is similar in echogenicity to the:
   a. kidney
   b. liver
   c. gut
   d. stomach

10. Herniation of the midgut resolves by week:
    a. 8
    b. 10
    c. 12
    d. 14

11. Complete situs inversus means the:
    a. cardiac apex is on the left and liver on the right
    b. cardiac apex is on right and liver on left
    c. cardiac apex is on the left and liver on the left
    d. cardiac apex is on the right and liver on the right

12. Duodenal atresia involves a fluid-filled stomach and duodenum at the site of obstruction, which demonstrates a(n):
    a. image of a small stomach
    b. "double-bubble" image
    c. elongated stomach image
    d. a long hypoechoic tubular appearance displaying the stomach and intestine without stricture

13. The descending colon wall-to-wall diameter measurement varies with fetal gestational age, but should not measure greater than _____ in a preterm fetus.
    a. 8 mm
    b. 14 mm
    c. 1.6 cm
    d. 2.0 cm

14. Mean fluid volume of amniotic fluid in a 20 week is:
    a. 250 mL
    b. 500 mL
    c. 750 mL
    d. 1,000 mL

15. Oligohydramnios is common with:
    a. renal anomalies
    b. cardiac anomalies
    c. thorax anomalies
    d. GI malformations

16. Single umbilical artery is usually insignificant, but is mostly associated with all except:
    a. gastrointestinal tract abnormalities
    b. renal and cardiac abnormalities
    c. increased incidence of trisomy
    d. pulmonary anomalies

17. Gastroschisis is a wall defect that typically occurs ____ the umbilical cord insertion.
    a. superior to
    b. inferior to
    c. to the left of
    d. to the right of

18. Ultrasound displays the fetal liver echotexture as:
    a. heterogeneous
    b. homogeneous
    c. hypointense
    d. hyperintense

Fill-in-the-Blank

1. Fetal abdominal organs have attained their normal adult position and structure in the early _____ trimester.

2. The presence of intact skin surface covering vertebral bodies is helpful to rule out _____.

3. The fetal abdominal wall displays an outer _____ genic skin line and a deeper, 1- to 3-mm _____ echoic muscular layer.

4. A two-vessel cord is most common in a _____ pregnancy.

5. An abdominal circumference should be obtained at the level of the junction of the umbilical vein, _____, and fetal _____.

6. Absence of the fetal gallbladder may be associated with biliary _____.

7. Filling and emptying of the fetal stomach occur causing absent stomach images, which requires _____ by a sonographer.

8. Midgut herniation is seen on an early fetus at the _____ portion of the embryo.

9. Duodenal atresia is the failure of the duodenum to change from a solid _____ of tissue during development to a _____.

10. A _____ is an obstruction caused by the bowel twisting upon its blood supply.

11. Meconium ileus is most often owing to _____.

12. The umbilical cord consists of _____ umbilical vein and _____ umbilical arteries.

13. Echogenic bowel can be associated with swallowed _____.

14. An omphalocele has a _____ whereas gastroschisis does not.

15. Midgut volvulus is usually diagnosed in the first days of life; the infant typically presents with _____.

16. The internal structures of the fetal kidneys are not reliably assessed before _____ weeks.

17. Esophageal maldevelopment is mostly related to the _____ gender.

18. An echogenic mass within the fetal gallbladder may be related to _____ or _____.

19. Diffuse liver calcifications occur in fetuses with intrauterine _____, especially those caused by pathogens responsible for _____ infections.

20. Oligohydramnios and the stress of nonimmune hydrops may result in the physiologic absence of _____ fluid.

Short Answer

1. Explain why the distal small bowel does not demonstrate filling until the third trimester.

2. Duodenal atresia is often related to multiple anomalies. State the associated anomalies.

3. Echogenic appearing bowel may be caused by a normal fetal abdominal process. It may also be a cause of concern. Explain.

4. List the three most common fetal bowel obstructions.

IMAGE EVALUATION/PATHOLOGY

Review the images and answer the following questions.

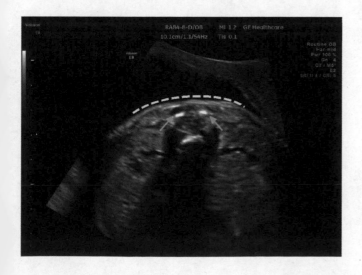

1. a. Name the view and the state of what is shown.
   b. Name the structures the arrows are directed toward.

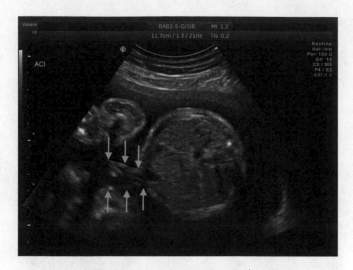

2. Explain the anatomy the arrows are directed toward.

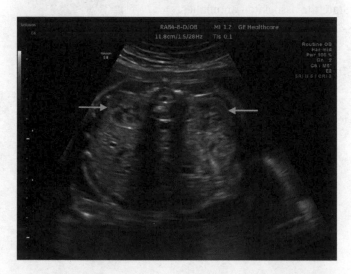

3. Name the anatomy the arrows are pointing toward.

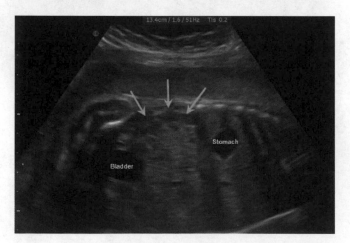

4. What are the arrows directed toward?

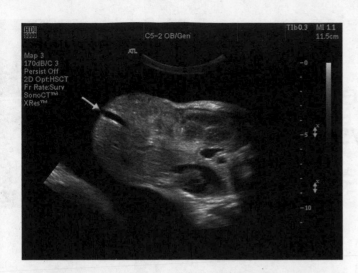

5. Diagnose this fetal image.

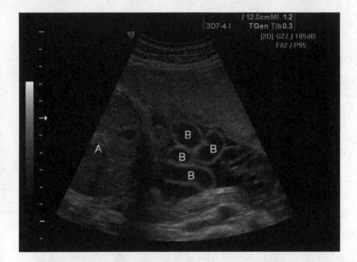

6. Diagnose the fetal image. A, abdomen; B, bowel.

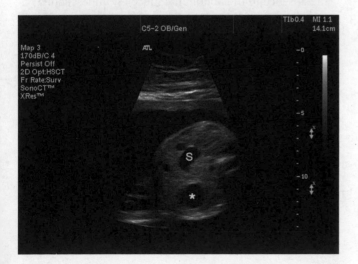

7. Explain the reason that two well-circumscribed hypoechoic structures are visualized in the fetal abdomen.

CHAPTER 28

Sonographic Assessment of the Fetal Genitourinary System and Fetal Pelvis

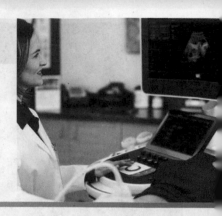

REVIEW OF GLOSSARY TERMS

Matching

Matching the key terms with their definitions.

KEY TERMS

1. _____ agenesis

2. _____ aplasia

3. _____ bladder exstrophy

4. _____ caliectasis

5. _____ dysmorphism

6. _____ horseshoe kidney

7. _____ hydrocele

8. _____ HASTE

9. _____ hypoplasia

10. _____ posterior urethral valves

11. _____ Potter sequence

12. _____ prune belly syndrome

13. _____ 3D imaging

14. _____ hydronephrosis

DEFINITIONS

a. Serous fluid accumulation in a body cavity such as the scrotum

b. Representing two genders

c. Underdevelopment or incomplete development of a body part

d. This group of findings, also called Potter syndrome or oligohydramnios sequence, includes renal conditions such as agenesis, obstructive processes, and acquired or inherited cystic disease.

e. Complete absence of a body part

f. Type of kidney where the upper poles fuse resulting in an appearance similar to a horseshoe

g. Congenital disorder of the urinary system resulting in the absence of the abdominal muscles, undescended testicles, and urinary tract problems

h. Congenital anomaly where the bladder is outside the body through a ventral wall defect inferior to the umbilical cord

i. Dilation of the renal pelvices and calyces, usually caused by obstruction

j. Failure of development

k. Obstructing membrane in the male urethra located posteriorly owing to abnormal urethral development

l. Dilation of the renal calyces

m. Half-Fourier acquisition single-shot turbo spine-echo; a fast spin method to obtain the MRI data set

n. From a volume data set, static 3D images can display height, width, and depth of anatomy (three dimensions) from any orthogonal plane.

CHAPTER REVIEW

Multiple Choice

Complete each question by circling the best answer.

1. In the first trimester, fetal kidneys appear _____ to the surrounding anatomy.
   a. hypoechoic
   b. isoechoic
   c. hyperechoic
   d. echogenic

2. When the second-trimester fetal renals are difficult to visualize, what method will assist in imaging them?
   a. Repositioning the mother
   b. Giving the mother 20 ounces of water to drink
   c. Color and/or power Doppler
   d. Reimaging the region after the fetus moves

3. The fetal bladder should be visualized by:
   a. 7 to 9 weeks
   b. 9 to 11 weeks
   c. 11 to 13 weeks
   d. 13 to 15 weeks

4. The fetal bladder fills and voids approximately once every:
   a. 15 minutes
   b. 30 minutes
   c. 60 minutes
   d. 2 hours

5. Bladder wall thickness cannot be visualized clearly without:
   a. a completely voided structure
   b. the bladder being distended
   c. a transverse approach
   d. ascites

6. Oligohydramnios is defined as an amniotic fluid volume of less than ____ cc, as indicated by a maximum vertical pocket (MVP) of less than 2 cm or an amniotic fluid index (AFI) of less than ____ cm on ultrasound.
   a. 500, 5
   b. 750, 5
   c. 500, 2
   d. 750, 2

7. _____ is a condition that a fetus has pulmonary hypoplasia secondary to oligohydramnios, typically owing to renal failure.
   a. Prune belly syndrome
   b. VUR
   c. Hirschsprung disease
   d. Potter syndrome

8. In the case of the unilateral agenesis, the existing kidney is invariably larger than in a fetus with two kidneys owing to:
   a. compensatory hypertrophy
   b. anhydramnios
   c. double renal artery in the existing kidney
   d. UPJ

9. Renal ectopia is a condition:
   a. that is incompatible with life
   b. where the bilateral kidneys are cystic
   c. of aplastic kidneys
   d. where a kidney is positioned outside of the renal fossa

10. Horseshoe kidney has the highest prevalence in fetuses with:
    a. Turner syndrome
    b. Down syndrome
    c. Edwards syndrome
    d. Patau syndrome

11. Severe fetal hydronephrosis is an APRPD over:
    a. 9 mm
    b. 11 mm
    c. 13 mm
    d. 15 mm

12. The prognosis is poor for a fetus with all except:
    a. bilateral hydronephrosis
    b. pulmonary hypoplasia
    c. isoechoic renal echogenicity
    d. bladder obstruction

13. In a 30-week fetus, megaureter is diagnosed when the ureter measures greater than:
    a. 3 mm
    b. 5 mm
    c. 6 mm
    d. 7 mm

14. A ureterocele is mostly associated with:
    a. a duplicated collecting system
    b. bilateral ureters
    c. a distended bladder
    d. males

15. Predominantly female renal and/or bladder anomalies include:
    a. crossed renal ectopia
    b. obstructive uropathy
    c. polycystic kidneys
    d. Prune belly syndrome

16. Causes for UPJ include all except:
    a. ureteral kinks
    b. peripelvic adhesions
    c. aberrant crossing renal vessels
    d. bladder dilation

17. Mesoblastic nephromas are mostly:
    a. related to oligohydramnios
    b. related to polyhydramnios
    c. related to a poor prognosis
    d. small

18. The fetal adrenals are best imaged in the:
    a. first trimester
    b. second trimester
    c. third trimester
    d. any trimester

19. Labels relating to disorders of sex development include all except:
    a. sex chromosome genotype
    b. pseudo-hermaphroditism
    c. ambiguous genitalia
    d. intersex

20. Choose the type of kidney that causes hypertension.
    a. Echogenic
    b. Enlarged
    c. Pelvic
    d. Horseshoe

Fill-in-the-Blank

1. The most common fetal malformation involves the _____ system.

2. In a transverse plane, fetal kidneys are _____ shaped.

3. The _____ arteries will assist in locating the fetal bladder.

4. The amount of amniotic fluid observed has a direct correlation to the _____ of the fetus.

5. The presence of _____ after 16 weeks' gestation raises suspicion for a malfunctioning GU system.

6. Renal _____ is the congenital absence of one or both kidneys.

7. _____ renal ectopia is a kidney located on the opposite side from which its ureter inserts into the bladder.

8. A pelvic kidney is located _____ to the renal fossa and _____ to the bladder.

9. Pelvic dilation in the third trimester means the renal pelvis is dilated over _____.

10. _____ is the permanent or intermittent retrograde flow of urine from the bladder into the upper urinary tract.

11. Autosomal recessive polycystic kidney disease (ARPKD) affects both kidneys and is also known as _____ polycystic kidney disease.

12. A single, nonseptated renal cyst with well-defined borders and no communication between the renal pelvis describes a _____ renal cyst.

13. The most basic conventional grading system for hydronephrosis characterizes the kidneys as _____, _____, or _____.

14. Bladder exstrophy demonstrates as a soft tissue mass extending from the _____ wall, with nonvisualization of the normal fetal bladder.

15. _____ kidneys are the most common renal fusion anomaly.

16. A posterior urethral valve is an obstructing _____ in the posterior urethra caused by redundant membranous folds.

17. The most common cause of congenital obstructive hydronephrosis is _____ obstruction.

18. _____ is the failure of the testes to complete the migratory descent into the scrotum.

19. Megacystitis is _____.

20. Pelviectasis is dilation of the _____ and _____.

Short Answer

1. Explain common ovarian anomalies that can be seen sonographically in the female fetus.

2. Name and explain the condition demonstrating two commonly seen umbilical arteries in the fetal pelvis without a cystic structure in between them.

3. Compare and contrast caliectasis, pelviectasis, and pelvicaliectasis.

IMAGE EVALUATION/PATHOLOGY

Review the images and answer the following questions.

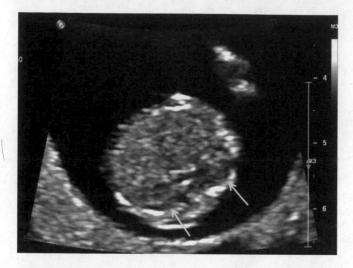

1. a. What are the arrows directed toward?
   b. Are the structures normal?
   c. Describe the central portion of the structure.
   d. Name the view.

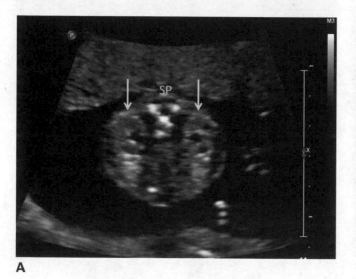

A

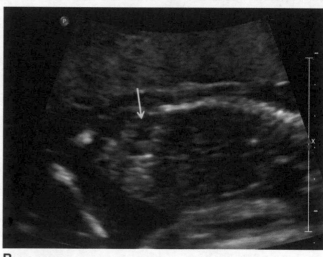

B

2. a. Image A is a transverse demonstrating bilateral kidneys (K); image B is a coronal view of the same fetus. Both images show an arrow. What structure is the arrow pointing at?
   b. Name the anomaly.

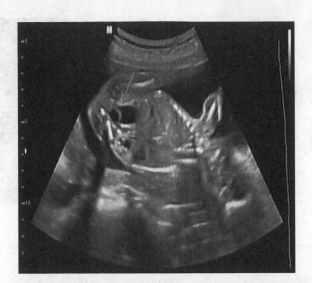

3. Explain the anomaly seen in this 22-week fetal bladder indicated by arrow.

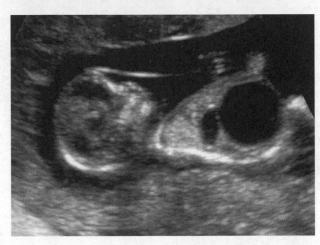

4. Name the two hypoechoic structures in the sagittal fetus.

CHAPTER 29

Normal and Abnormal Fetal Limbs

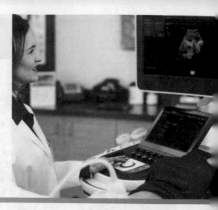

REVIEW OF GLOSSARY TERMS

Matching

Match the key terms with their definitions.

KEY TERMS

1. _____ mesomelia

2. _____ syndactyly

3. _____ talipes

4. _____ rhizomelia

5. _____ acromelia

6. _____ platyspondyly

7. _____ polydactyly

8. _____ micromelia

DEFINITIONS

a. Shortening of the most proximal portion of a fetal limb
b. Abnormally short limb
c. Flattened vertebral bodies with a decreased distance between the endplates
d. Fusion of soft tissue or body segments of fetal digits
e. Shortening of the most distal position of a fetal limb
f. Condition of having more than the normal number of digits on a hand or foot
g. Abnormal shortening of the middle portion of a limb
h. Abnormal position of the fetal foot and ankle

CHAPTER REVIEW

Multiple Choice

Complete each question by circling the best answer.

1. Between 32 and 35 weeks, the epiphyseal region of the _____ can be seen sonographically:
   a. radius and ulna
   b. tibia and fibula
   c. humerus
   d. femur

2. The normal fetal hand should be viewed in:
   a. a flexed position
   b. an extended position
   c. both flexion and extension positions
   d. fixed position

3. A short limb dysplasia affecting the humerus is:
   a. rhizomelia
   b. osteogenesis imperfecta
   c. camptomelia
   d. achondrogenesis

4. Shortening of an entire limb is known as:
   a. hypophosphatasia
   b. micromelia
   c. mesomelia
   d. dysplasia

5. Micrognathia is:
   a. an abnormally small lower jaw
   b. abnormally shaped ears
   c. frontal bossing
   d. a prominent forehead

6. A type of skeletal dysplasia demonstrating sonographically as a narrow bell-shaped thorax is most likely:
   a. pulmonary hypoplasia
   b. VACTERL
   c. OI Type IV dysplasia
   d. short rib syndrome

7. Characteristics of rhizomelic limb bowing, frontal bossing, a low nasal bridge, a "trident" configuration of the hand, with possible macrocephaly, and hydrocephaly may be noted in:
   a. achondrogenesis
   b. achondroplasia
   c. sirenomelia
   d. phocomelia

8. Select the syndrome with the best prognosis for living into adulthood.
   a. Asphyxiating thoracic dysplasia
   b. Thanatophoric dysplasia
   c. Achondrogenesis
   d. Ellis-van Creveld Syndrome (EvC)

9. Central polydactyly affects the:
   a. radial side of the hand
   b. ulnar side of the hand
   c. three middle digits of the hand
   d. thumb

10. The absence of one or more hands is:
    a. phocomelia
    b. hemimelia
    c. apodia
    d. acheiria

11. Holt-Oram syndrome demonstrates abnormalities of the skeletal system and:
    a. respiratory system
    b. cardiac system
    c. cranium
    d. urinary system

12. Amniotic band sequence is believed to be related to all except:
    a. cleft lip/palate
    b. ectopia cordis
    c. polydactyly
    d. amputation

13. The "mermaid syndrome" is a rare and lethal and also known as:
    a. absent radii syndrome
    b. sirenomelia
    c. mesomelia
    d. congenital hypophosphatasia

14. Fetal hands and feet anomalies include all but:
    a. extra fingers
    b. clubbing
    c. ischemia
    d. finger reduction

15. Congenital hypophosphatasia is an inherited disease related to:
    a. defective bone mineralization
    b. maternal cocaine use
    c. maternal diabetes
    d. amniotic sheeting

16. Maternal hyperthyroidism contributes to:
    a. phocomelia
    b. craniosynostosis
    c. caudal regression
    d. limb measurements below the 10th percentile

17. What is the most likely cause of digit and limb amputation?
    a. Amniotic sheets
    b. Oligohydramnios
    c. Amniotic bands
    d. Dysostosis

18. The most common cause of skeletal deformities is:
    a. oligohydramnios
    b. uterine tumor
    c. müllerian anomalies
    d. toxic agents

19. Polyhydramnios is common with all except:
    a. camptomelic dysplasia
    b. TD
    c. short rib-polydactyly syndrome
    d. achondroplasia

20. Select the thickest extremity long bone:
    a. tibia
    b. ulna
    c. fibula
    d. radius

Fill-in-the-Blank

1. An amniotic sheet appears as a membranous pillar within the amniotic fluid and is characterized by a _____ that projects into the amniotic cavity.

2. Primary ossification centers of limbs are visualized at _____ weeks.

3. Long bone epiphysis visualizes by _____ weeks, helping in determination of fetal maturity.

4. Skeletal dysplasia is the abnormal development of the _____ and osseous tissues.

5. The premature fusion of one or several cranial sutures is _____.

6. _____ is a condition characterized by abnormal ossification.

7. A dysplasia with an extremely poor prognosis owing to respiratory complications from hypoplastic lungs and micrognathia is _____.

8. OI (osteogenesis imperfecta) is rare, inheritable, and related to defects in _____ quality or quantity.

9. Meromelia is a(n) _____ of part of a limb.

10. A fetal forearm with an absent radius is frequently noted to have a radially deviated hand that appears as a _____.

11. VACTERL association is defined as: _____, _____, _____, _____, _____, _____.

12. Club foot is frequently caused by _____ or other conditions that limit fetal movement.

13. Amniotic bands, known as _____, are associated with medical procedures involving the uterine _____ and intrauterine infections.

14. Lower extremity fusion is postulated to be caused by a _____ steal phenomenon.

15. Skeletal dysplasias are mostly _____ to the fetus.

16. Osteogenesis imperfecta causes prenatal bone _____ and fractures.

17. A fetus with an extremely narrow thorax, rhizomelic limbs, polydactyly, pelvic anomalies, and renal anomalies describes _____ dysplasia.

18. Achondrogenesis is lethal because of _____.

19. The femur bone may resemble the _____ bone on fetal sonography.

20. On average, the fetal femur grows ___ mm a week up to 27 weeks, slowing to ____ mm per week for the rest of gestation.

Short Answer

1. Which fetal bony structures can be accurately measured to determine growth and size?

2. List the information that may be gathered from long bone measurements and evaluation.

3. Explain cranial abnormalities that are visualized with sonography interrogation.

4. Discuss the challenges of detecting and diagnosing skeletal dysplasia.

IMAGE EVALUATION/PATHOLOGY

Review the images and answer the following questions.

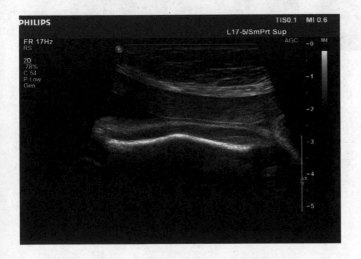

1. Name the structure in the image. Diagnose the condition.

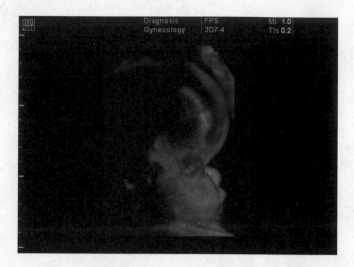

2. What type of imaging produced the image? Describe the visualized structure and position. State the anomaly.

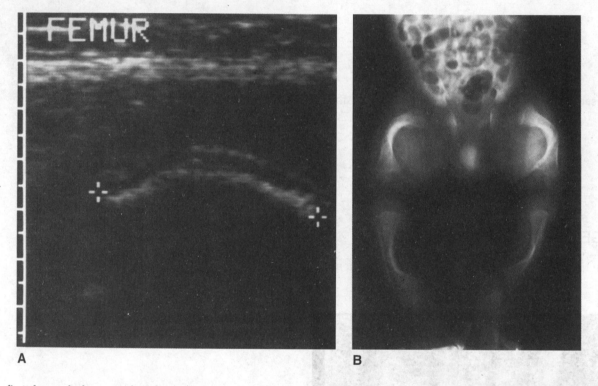

A

B

3. Define the pathology on the ultrasound in image A and the radiograph in image B and make a diagnosis.

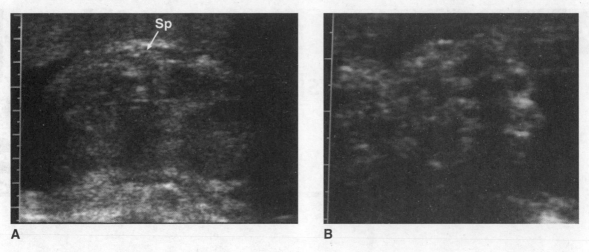

A   Sp

B

4. Explain the syndrome based on the transverse view of the fetal spine in image A and magnified view of the fetal hand in image B.

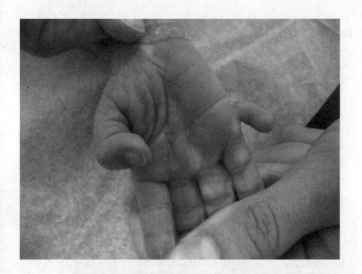

5. Identify and label the extremity anomaly.

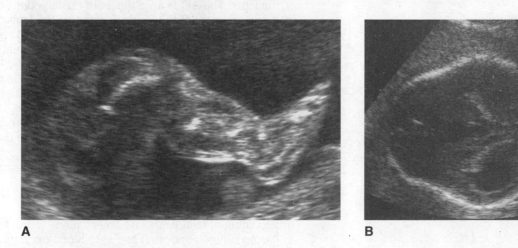

A

B

6. Name the type of dysplasia the two images depict.

CHAPTER 30

The Biophysical Profile

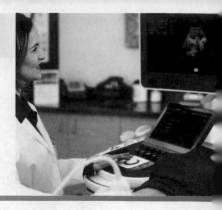

REVIEW OF GLOSSARY TERMS

Matching

Match the key terms with their definitions.

KEY TERMS

1. _____ hypoxemia

2. _____ pH

3. _____ amniotic fluid index (AFI)

4. _____ asphyxia

5. _____ false negative

6. _____ biophysical profile (BPP)

7. _____ oxytocin challenge test (OCT)

8. _____ nonstress test (NST)

9. _____ cardiotocography (CTG)

10. _____ false positive

11. _____ acidosis

12. _____ amniotic fluid volume (AFV)

13. _____ hypercapnia

14. _____ modified biophysical profile (mBPP)

15. _____ oligohydramnios

DEFINITIONS

a. Incorrect negative test result when the state being tested is present; example: The fetus reacts during a BPP; however, there is fetal compromise owing to acidosis.

b. Low fluid surrounding the fetus

c. Abnormally high level of circulating carbon dioxide

d. Reduced blood oxygen levels

e. Prenatal testing including only the NST and AFI

f. Positive result when the state being tested is absent. Example: Nonreactive BPP owing to fetal sleep cycles

g. Intravenous injection of oxytocin causing the uterus to contract. Monitoring of the fetal reaction to uterine contractions aims to determine how the fetus reacts to environmental stress

h. Measure of alkalinity or acidity of the blood with neutral at 7; >7 is alkaline; <7 is acidic

i. Amount of fluid within the amniotic sac surrounding the fetus. The AFI is an estimate of this amount.

j. Rough estimate of the fluid surrounding the fetus obtained through the measurement of four pockets of amniotic fluid, one from each of the abdominal quadrants

k. Monitoring of fetal activity to include breathing movements, discrete movements, tone, and fluid surrounding the fetus accompanied by an NST

l. Blood pH <7 owing to an increase in hydrogen concentrations caused by impaired blood supply to the fetus

m. Technique of concurrently recording the fetal heartbeat and contractions

n. Decrease in oxygen content of the blood accompanied by an increase in carbon dioxide

o. Recording of fetal heart rate accelerations (normal) or decelerations (abnormal) owing to blood oxygen level changes resulting from uterine contractions

ANATOMY AND PHYSIOLOGY REVIEW

Image Labeling

Complete the labels in the images that follow.

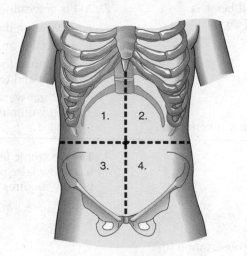

AFI quadrants

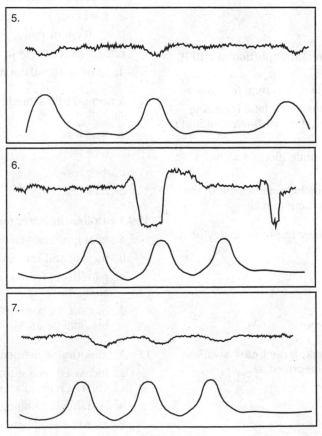

Decelerations

CHAPTER REVIEW

Multiple Choice

Complete each question by circling the best answer.

1. Ultrasound observance of fetal well-being is determined by all of the following except:
   a. body movements
   b. urine output
   c. spontaneous breathing
   d. heart decelerations

2. Electronic fetal heart rate monitoring is performed by:
   a. calculating AFV
   b. OCT
   c. BPP testing
   d. calculating fetal growth ratios

3. A fetal biophysical profile in utero observation includes all except:
   a. NST
   b. fetal tone
   c. fetal breathing
   d. gross body movements

4. In order to pass the fetal breathing portion of a BPP, the fetus must exhibit:
   a. breath-to-breath intervals of less than 6 seconds
   b. at least one episode of sustained fetal breathing of at least 30 seconds duration within a 30-minute span
   c. breathing episodes to include hiccups within a 30-minute interval
   d. spontaneous motion to include movement of the chest wall and of the abdominal wall

5. Fetal movements in pregnancy imply normalcy of the fetal:
   a. respiratory system
   b. musculoskeletal system
   c. CNS
   d. cerebrospinal fluid volume

6. Fetal movements of the trunk, large limbs, swallowing, face, and hands are categorized as:
   a. motion mode
   b. AFV
   c. tone
   d. gross body movements

7. AFI is determined by:
   a. measuring the deepest pocket of amniotic fluid
   b. subjective analysis
   c. measuring four quadrants in the deepest vertical pocket and totaling the values
   d. four transverse depth measurements of amniotic fluid within the pregnant uterus, summed and totaled

8. The electronic fetal heart monitoring method that has a low false positive, low false negative and usually requires several hours to complete is:
   a. OCT
   b. NST
   c. BPP
   d. AFI

9. Oligohydramnios is diagnosed when the amniotic fluid in four quadrants measures:
   a. 5.0 cm or less
   b. 19.0 cm or more
   c. less than 5.0 cm in a quadrant
   d. more than 9.0 cm in a quadrant

10. A normal BPP score is 8 or 10. An equivocal score is:
    a. 8 or less
    b. 6 or less
    c. 4 or less
    d. 2 or less

11. A cardiotachometer records:
    a. fetal gross movement
    b. uterine and cervical contractions
    c. patterns of fetal heart rate including baseline and changes
    d. blood flow patterns and Doppler assessment of the fetal heart

12. Acceleration is defined as:
    a. increased fetal gross body movement and tone involving more than six movements in 15 minutes
    b. sustained breathing beyond 60 seconds
    c. an AFI over 22 cm
    d. increase of the fetal heart rate over the baseline of at least 15 beats per minute, and lasting at least 15 seconds associated with fetal movement

13. Startle means:

    a. slow and small shifting of the fetal contour

    b. quick, generalized movement always initiated in limbs and sometimes spreading to neck and trunk

    c. regular in rate and amplitude

    d. irregular, intermittent, large-amplitude breaths; short duration of individual breaths

14. Normal fetal tone is:

    a. three flexion to extension movements with full return in a 30-minute span

    b. seen with movement of the extremities in a longitudinal fashion

    c. at least one episode of extension of extremities with return to position of flexion, or extension of spine with return to position of flexion is visualized in the 30-minute observation period

    d. three rolling movements of the trunk or long bones in a 30-minute observation period

15. An AFI plus an NST is known as:

    a. partial BPP

    b. modified BPP

    c. BPP – NST

    d. BPP

16. Regular patterns of fetal breathing are defined as:

    a. crescendo-decrescendo changes in rate and amplitude

    b. 40 to 60 breaths per minute

    c. intermittent, large-amplitude breaths

    d. observed in the 20- to 26-week fetus

17. BPP, AFI, and NST testing typically occurs:

    a. daily

    b. every other day

    c. twice weekly

    d. once weekly

18. Independent limb movements occur at:

    a. the 8th week

    b. the 9th week

    c. weeks 10 to 12

    d. the 14th week

19. Fetal movement is mostly related to:

    a. placental location

    b. AFV

    c. fetal individuality

    d. maturation of the CNS

20. Fetal breathing can be gauged with a real-time scanner by viewing the fetal abdomen in a longitudinal fashion, as well as by observing:

    a. abdominal contractions

    b. caudal–cephalad kidney movement

    c. sustained lower extremity flexion extension with pressure onto the anterior abdomen

    d. prolonged wide opening of jaws, followed by quick closure

Fill-in-the-Blank

1. Monitoring the fetus in the second and third trimesters can be performed by the mother in the way of

    _____.

2. _____, a decrease in oxygen content of the blood accompanied by an increase in carbon dioxide, can be evaluated by antepartum testing.

3. Two electronic fetal monitoring tests involving heart rate are _____ and _____.

4. The first maternal perception of fetal movement is known as _____.

5. AFI is determined by measuring depth of fluid of _____ quadrants.

6. Amniotic fluid cannot be measured in a pocket that contains _____.

7. The biophysical profile variables can earn a score of _____ if normal and a score of _____ if abnormal or do not meet the criteria.

8. Breathing movements increase during periods of _____, but decrease with maternal _____.

9. Fetal movement is usually noted by the mother at _____ weeks.

10. A fetal reactive NST is defined as _____ accelerations with a _____-minute span.

11. An increase of the fetal heart rate over the baseline of at least 10 beats per minute and lasting at least 10 seconds is considered normal for fetuses _____ weeks gestation.

12. The term _____ is applied to an NST that did not respond as expected in the allotted time span.

13. Jerky contractions of the diaphragm or abrupt consistent displacement of the diaphragm, thorax, and abdomen are _____.

14. The _____ plane through the fetal chest best demonstrates fetal breathing.

15. _____ stimulation results in a significant reduction in the number of nonreactive NSTs and a decrease in the time required for a reactive test to occur.

16. A nonreactive fetus may respond to maternal _____, _____ stimulation, _____ manipulation of the maternal abdomen, and _____ ingestion to stimulate or awaken them.

17. It has been noted that at 20 weeks the fetal heart rate increases with fetal _____.

18. Hiccups are caused by a contraction of the _____.

19. During maternal hypoxemia, cessation of fetal _____ occurs.

20. Rhythmic bursts of regular jaw opening and closing at a rate of about one per second suggests _____ activity.

Short Answer

1. Describe fetal movement and compare it with fetal tone. Explain the variable requirements in order to obtain a score of 2.

2. When is antenatal testing for fetal asphyxia performed and why?

3. In what order do BPP variables usually become abnormal?

4. Why is it important to obtain a thorough maternal history prior to diagnosing a BPP, NST, or OCT?

5. How does pH correlate to BPP?

IMAGE EVALUATION/PATHOLOGY

Review the images and answer the following questions.

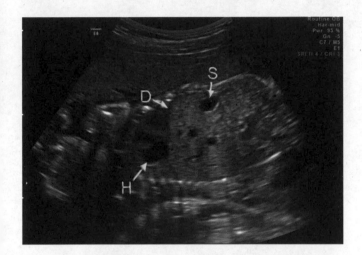

1. Identify the view and anatomy depicted with a "D,"
"H," and "S." Correlate the view with a BPP examination and state the value of the image when seen in
real time.

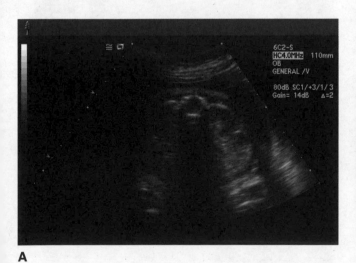

A

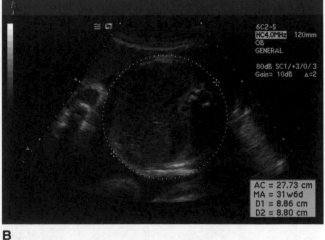

B

2. Explain the view, anatomy, and information of both images to include biometrics. Keep in mind that the fetus
rolled clockwise from image A to B and continued the rolling motions throughout the scan. What BPP knowledge
can be derived from this limited information?

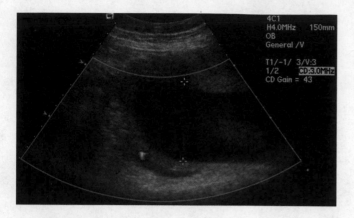

3. Discuss the image. What is the significance of color Doppler in the lower left of the image?

CHAPTER 31

Multiple Gestations

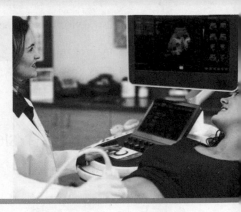

REVIEW OF GLOSSARY TERMS

Matching

Match the key terms with their definitions.

KEY TERMS

1. _____ follicle stimulating hormone (FSH)

2. _____ monoamniotic

3. _____ biometry

4. _____ nonimmune hydrops

5. _____ hypervolemic

6. _____ monozygotic

7. _____ amnionicity

8. _____ thermocoagulation

9. _____ gamete intrafallopian transfer (GIFT)

10. _____ in vitro fertilization (IVF)

11. _____ anembryonic

12. _____ quadruplet

13. _____ chorionicity

14. _____ oligohydramnios

15. _____ dizygotic

16. _____ zygote

17. _____ hysterotomy

18. _____ mortality

19. _____ polyhydramnios

DEFINITIONS

a. Surgical incision into the uterus, i.e., cesarean section

b. Mixing of the ovum and sperm within the fallopian tubes allowing for fertilization within the woman's body

c. Hormone that induces the growth of Graafian follicles

d. Increase in circulating blood volume

e. Injection of a sperm into the oocyte

f. Two zygotes as a result of the fertilization of two ova

g. Determination of the number of the fetal membranes called the amnion

h. Measurements done on an embryo or fetus such as a crown–rump length (CRL) or biparietal diameter (BPD)

i. Determination of the number of chorionic membranes adjacent to the uterus

j. Lack of an embryo

k. Large fetus that falls in the 90th percentile for weight

l. One zygote

m. Death rate owing to a specific disease

n. Low amniotic fluid levels

o. Four

p. Too much amniotic fluid

q. Use of heat to seal tissue

r. Fertilized ovum with 23 pairs of chromosomes

s. Fertilization of the ovum outside the uterus

t. One amnion

u. Incidence of disease

v. Edema, accumulation of fluid in tissues and in the peritoneal cavity, and chest, in a fetus not affected by erythroblastosis fetalis

w. Abundant

20. _____ intracytoplasmic sperm injection (ICSI)

21. _____ macrosomic

22. _____ plethoric

23. _____ morbidity

ANATOMY AND PHYSIOLOGY REVIEW

Image Labeling

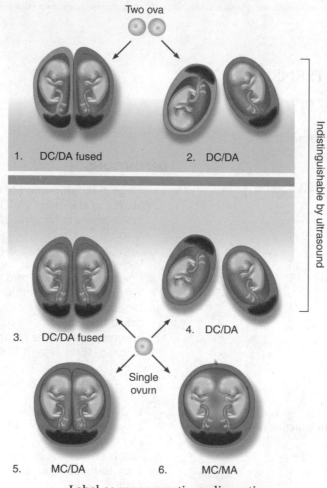

Label as monozygotic or dizygotic

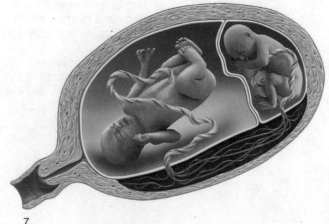

7.

Label the type of syndrome

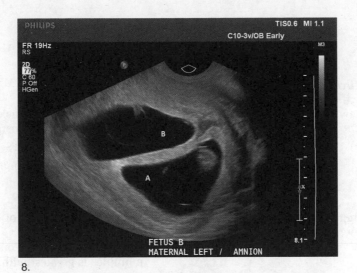

8.

Label the type of pregnancy

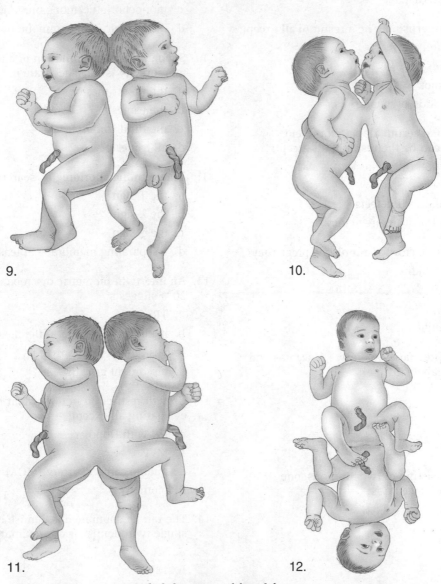

9.

10.

11.

12.

Label the types of fused fetuses

CHAPTER REVIEW

Multiple Choice

Complete each question by circling the best answer.

1. What is least related to twinning?
   a. Choriocarcinoma
   b. IUGR
   c. Preterm birth
   d. Fetal anomalies

2. Spontaneously occurring monozygotic twinning is noted to be influenced by:
   a. random factors
   b. economic status
   c. genetics
   d. advanced maternal age

3. A large for date uterus may be a result of all except:
   a. macrosomic fetus
   b. uterine fibroids
   c. oligohydramnios
   d. multiple gestation pregnancy

4. Increased maternal serum alpha-fetoprotein (MSAFP) levels can be the result of all except:
   a. fetal open neural tube defects
   b. placental masses
   c. fetal abdominal wall defects
   d. uterine fibroids during pregnancy

5. What is not a risk factor for a multiple pregnancy?
   a. Decreased morbidity
   b. IUGR
   c. TTTS
   d. Low birth weight

6. A monozygotic pregnancy with two placentas and two amnions is labeled:
   a. DC/DA
   b. DZ/MA
   c. MC/MA
   d. MZ/DA

7. A pregnancy consisting of two amnions, one chorion, and one placenta is:
   a. DC/DA
   b. DC/MA
   c. MC/DA
   d. MC/MA

8. Preeclampsia, hypertension, placental abruption, placenta previa, and postpartum hemorrhage are:
   a. associated with TTTS
   b. maternal complications of a multiple gestation pregnancy
   c. risks of TRAP
   d. fetal complications of twinning

9. The risk of an adverse outcome or abnormality with multiples is greatest with:
   a. dichorionic/diamniotic twins
   b. monochorionic/diamniotic twins
   c. monochorionic/monoamniotic twins
   d. dichorionic/monoamniotic twins

10. Sonographic determination of chorionicity and amnionicity is most accurate in:
    a. the first trimester
    b. the trimester
    c. the third trimester
    d. all trimesters

11. To determine chorionicity, search for all except:
    a. the T sign
    b. the λ sign
    c. the Y sign
    d. a separating membrane at least 1.5 mm thick

12. An intertwin biometric discrepancy of more than 20% suggests:
    a. TRTS
    b. likelihood of gender difference
    c. positional variation
    d. discordant growth

13. Growth restriction in discordant twins is assessed by evaluating all except:
    a. UA with Doppler
    b. MVP
    c. middle cerebral artery (MCA) with Doppler
    d. biometry

14. The rate of spontaneous demise of singleton and single twin demise is approximately:
    a. 5%
    b. 12%
    c. 21%
    d. 32%

15. What is least likely to contribute to an adverse outcome with a twin pregnancy?
    a. A higher rate of cesarean section
    b. Age
    c. Preeclampsia
    d. Diabetes

16. A primary fetal risk factor for mortality and long-term morbidity with multiple gestations is:
    a. postpartum hemorrhage
    b. oligohydramnios
    c. discordant fetal position
    d. low birth weight

17. An abnormality revealing a normal twin combined with a poorly defined twin possessing an irregular or no cardiac structure is:
    a. TTTS
    b. TRAP sequence
    c. recipient syndrome
    d. donor syndrome

18. TRAP sequence is commonly referred to as:
    a. acardiac twinning
    b. pump twin
    c. hemodynamic dependency
    d. anastomoses

19. TTTS is associated with _____ cord insertion.
    a. eccentric
    b. peripheral
    c. central
    d. velamentous

20. Conjoined twins connecting at the thorax are classified as:
    a. pygopagus
    b. omphalopagus
    c. thoracopagus
    d. craniopagus

Fill-in-the-Blank

1. Twins of different sex originate from two separate _____ and are thus _____.

2. If two discrete placentas can be identified on ultrasound, the pregnancy must be _____.

3. Monozygotic twinning is the result of a _____ ovum.

4. Several authors have reported that the growth rates of normal multiples in the second and third trimesters follow that of singleton pregnancies until around _____ weeks.

5. Triplet or higher-order gestations, biometric parameters may start to lag sooner in pregnancy, except for _____, which seems to closely follow nomograms developed for singletons.

6. An _____ resistance to blood flow within the umbilical arteries (UA) or a _____ resistance observed in the MCAs may occur in the setting of IUGR.

7. Multiple gestation maternal complications include _____, _____, _____, _____, _____, _____, _____, and _____.

8. ART has been shown to increase the rate of fetal vessels overlying the cervical os, also known as _____.

9. Concordant defects in twins is mostly related to _____ twins.

10. Chorionicity and amnionicity determination utilizing ultrasound is most accurate in the _____ trimester.

11. An accurate and easy method of determining the type of twinning involves counting the number of _____ sacs.

12. The _____ sign refers to the presence of a triangular projection of placental tissue extending into the vase of the junction of two chorionic membranes.

13. In a twin pregnancy, fetuses measuring _____ or more days difference by CRL are considered discordant.

14. Conjoined twins are the result of the incomplete division of the embryo during the implantation stage occurring after day _____.

15. An early twin pregnancy that delivers a singleton fetus is known as a _____ pregnancy.

16. All multiple gestations should be considered _____ pregnancies.

17. A gestational sac lacking fetal membranes is a _____ pregnancy.

18. Periodically removing fluid from a twin polyhydramniotic sac is known as _____amniocentesis.

19. The highest risk form of twinning is _____.

20. Selective reduction should never be performed on a _____ pregnancy due to the risk of passing a _____ substance from demise twin into the surviving twin.

Short Answer

1. List complications of multiples in a pregnancy.

2. A 24-year-old G1 patient was recently diagnosed as DC/DA. She is excited and curious about the twins and requests an explanation of her pregnancy.

3. Explain the zygote division timeline associated with monozygotic twinning.

4. Discuss the finding of one gestational sac versus two gestational sacs in a transvaginal first-trimester ultrasound.

5. State methods of identifying twins on follow-up ultrasound examinations.

IMAGE EVALUATION/PATHOLOGY

Review the images and answer the following questions.

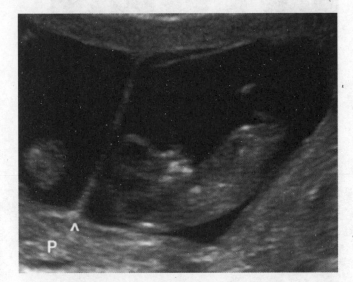

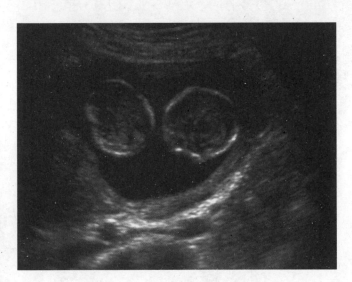

1. What type of "sign" does the amniotic membrane show?

2. Name the type of pregnancy.

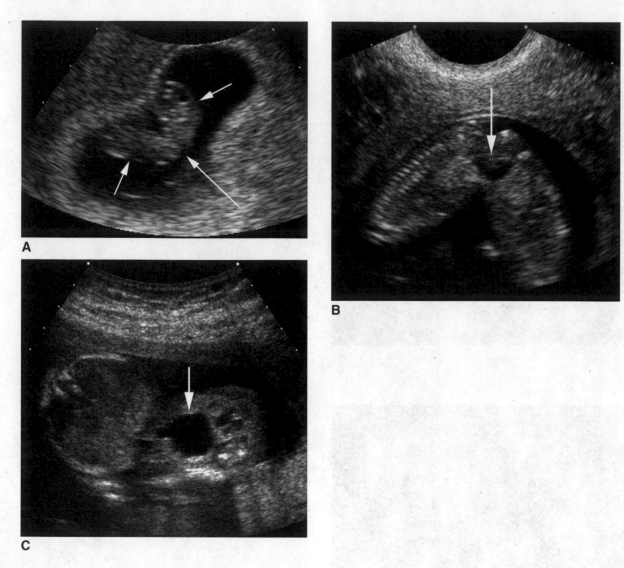

A

B

C

3. Describe and diagnose this type of pregnancy.

CHAPTER 32

Fetal Growth Restriction

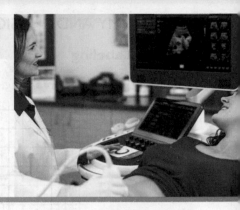

REVIEW OF GLOSSARY TERMS

Matching

Match the key terms with their definitions.

KEY TERMS

1. _____ small for gestational age (SGA)

2. _____ analyte

3. _____ sensitivity

4. _____ placental mosaicism

5. _____ hypoxemia

6. _____ low birth weight (LBW)

7. _____ nonstress test (NST)

8. _____ trisomy

9. _____ preeclampsia

10. _____ idiopathic

11. _____ morbidity

12. _____ biophysical profile (BPP)

13. _____ specificity

14. _____ Doppler velocimetry

15. _____ oligohydramnios

16. _____ aneuploidy

17. _____ fetal growth restriction (FGR) or intrauterine growth restriction (IUGR)

18. _____ mortality

DEFINITIONS

a. Hypertension and protein in the urine, occurring during pregnancy

b. Without known cause

c. Having three copies of a specific chromosome

d. Chemical substance that is the subject of analysis

e. Abnormal chromosome number

f. Combined observation of four separate fetal biophysical variables (fetal breathing movements, fetal body movement, fetal tone, amniotic fluid index) obtained via ultrasound. This can be done with or without an NST (8-point or 10-point BPP).

g. Birth weight below 2,500 g or 5 lbs 8 oz

h. Noninvasive ultrasound test that assesses blood flow velocity profiles from which indices of impedance can be obtained or flow volumes can be calculated

i. Incidence of a specific disease in a population for a set amount of time

j. Diagnosis used to describe an infant who is smaller than expected for the gestational age

k. The proportion of people who test negative for the disease to those who do not have the disease

l. Low amniotic fluid levels

m. Estimated fetal weight or abdominal circumference <10th percentile for gestational age

n. Condition characterized by the discrepancy between the chromosomal makeup of the fetus and placenta

o. Frequency of deaths in a specific population

p. The proportion of people who test positive for a disease to those who actually have the disease

q. Low oxygen blood level

r. Method of assessing fetal well-being by observing the fetal heart rate accelerations

ANATOMY AND PHYSIOLOGY REVIEW

Image Labeling

Complete the labels in the images that follow.

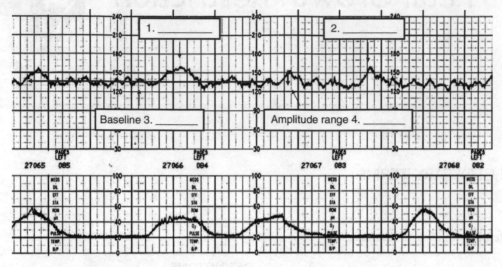

Nonstress test

1. and 2. What do the arrows point to?

3. Name the baseline heart rate.

4. What is the amplitude range of the fetal heart rate?

CHAPTER REVIEW

Multiple Choice

Complete each question by circling the best answer.

1. Conditions such as poor maternal weight gain, previous FGR infant, maternal complications, and inadequate symphysis to fundal height growth are suggestive of:
   a. LBW
   b. macrosomic fetus
   c. FGR
   d. idiopathic anomalies

2. Select the description that does not characterize FGR.
   a. Growth 2 SD below the mean for gestational age
   b. Fetal lagging abdominal circumference
   c. An EFW <10th percentile
   d. Macrosomia

3. A cause of intrauterine growth restriction is:
   a. maternal hypertension
   b. incorrect LMP
   c. unexpected ovulation date
   d. small parents

4. FGR affects the fetal blood flow by:
   a. increasing cardiac output
   b. redistributing it to the fetal brain
   c. redistributing it to the fetal liver
   d. an increase in umbilical vein volume

5. FGR can cause poor health for the fetus into adulthood. They include all except:
   a. hypertension
   b. diabetes
   c. anorexia
   d. obesity

6. Preeclampsia:
   a. is a condition where elevated protein is discovered in the maternal urine
   b. is a condition of low blood pressure
   c. causes maternal hydronephrosis owing to elevated urinary protein
   d. causes fetal weight gain

7. A common cause of FGR is:

    a. thyroid insufficiency

    b. uterine structure

    c. placental abnormalities

    d. elevated liver enzymes

8. Herpes simplex virus, cytomegalovirus, rubella, and varicella zoster are _____ which relate to fetal growth restriction.

    a. chromosomal conditions

    b. enzymes

    c. functional conditions

    d. infectious conditions

9. Atypical growth pattern where the fetal AC lags the BPD, HC, and FL is known as:

    a. symmetric

    b. FGR/IUGR

    c. asymmetric

    d. <10th percentile

10. Congenital malformation, drugs, and chromosomal abnormalities are usually responsible for:

    a. stage II birth defects

    b. symmetric FGR/IUGR

    c. asymmetric FGR/IUGR

    d. Stage I hospital admissions

11. Identification of growth-restricted fetuses is done through sonographic EFW, fundal height, and:

    a. serum analytes

    b. fetal urinalysis

    c. CMP

    d. maternal urinalysis

12. BPP should only be performed when:

    a. the fetus is 22 weeks or more

    b. the fetus is in a vertex position

    c. 30 weeks or more

    d. delivery of the fetus would be considered

13. A fundal height measurement difference of more than __ cm less than expected after 20 weeks gestation is cause for suspicion of FGR.

    a. 2

    b. .5

    c. 3

    d. 1

14. If FGR is suspected, the ideal interval between growth evaluations is every:

    a. week

    b. 2 weeks

    c. 3 weeks

    d. 4 weeks

15. The predictive error of ultrasound _____ as the gestation increases.

    a. decreases

    b. remains the same

    c. does not change

    d. increases

16. Common maternal treatments to increase growth in an FGR fetus includes all except:

    a. nonimpact exercise

    b. fish oil

    c. aspirin

    d. hyperoxygenation

17. A normal nonstress test displays:

    a. fetal tone

    b. two or more accelerations within 20 minutes

    c. fetal breathing

    d. amniotic fluid volume

18. Hypothermia, hematologic complications, and hypoglycemia are fetal conditions related to:

    a. preeclampsia

    b. FGR

    c. acidemia

    d. hypoxemia

19. FGR children, especially preterm, have an elevated risk of all except:

    a. low blood pressure

    b. behavioral problems

    c. inferior school performance

    d. neurological damage

20. Select the correct fetal category for a fetus displaying biometric parameters below 10% without a known cause, possibly relating to parental habitus and family history, small AC/BPD/HC/FL measurements, normal AFI, normal BPD/AC ratio, and normal placenta.

    a. Macrosomia

    b. Symmetrical FGR/IUGR

    c. Asymmetrical FGR/IUGR

    d. SGA

Fill-in-the-Blank

1. The fetus with poor intrauterine growth has an _____ risk for perinatal mortality compared with the normal size fetus.

2. Cord anomalies that increase the risk of FGR are _____ and _____.

3. FGR infants usually achieve normal growth at the age of _____.

4. Measurement of the largest pocket of fluid that is free of fetal parts or umbilical cord is called _____.

5. Poor intrauterine growth and subsequent LBW are common features of many _____ abnormalities.

6. The most common chromosomal abnormalities that increase a fetus's risk for FGR are _____ syndrome, _____ syndrome, and _____ syndrome.

7. There are over 50 published formulas for EFW. More recent publications show that the _____ formula is consistently better than other formulas.

8. The cause of FGR/IUGR may be idiopathic or _____.

9. A potentially concerning result from a BPP score is a score of _____ or less.

10. Maternal medical conditions that effect blood circulation result in a _____ in uteroplacental blood flow and can lead to FGR.

11. Maternal _____ in pregnancy is one of the leading causes of FGR.

12. Preeclampsia occurs during the _____ half of pregnancy.

13. In a normal fetus, the MCA is a _____ impedance circulation with continuous _____ flow.

14. _____ Doppler may help differentiate a constitutionally small fetus and a pathologic FGR fetus.

15. Risk factors or etiologies of FGR can be divided into three groups: _____, _____, and _____.

16. Estimated fetal _____, sonographic biometry, Doppler flow, and _____ fluid changes assist in identification of growth-restricted fetuses.

17. Avoiding and cessation of smoking during pregnancy can increase fetal _____.

18. Increased hypoxemia, arterial resistance, and nutritional deprivation lead to _____ dysfunction.

19. Fetal circulatory redistribution when there is placental dysfunction is termed _____.

20. Antenatal surveillance is done with four fetal growth assessments: _____, _____, _____, and _____.

Short Answer

1. Name three common sites that Doppler interrogates for anomalies in pregnancy.

2. Name placental risk factors related to FGR.

3. State fetal assessment protocols that are most commonly utilized in gauging fetal well-being once delivery is being considered.

4. Review and explain the fetal heart rate patterns noted in a nonstress test.

IMAGE EVALUATION/PATHOLOGY

Review the images and answer the following questions.

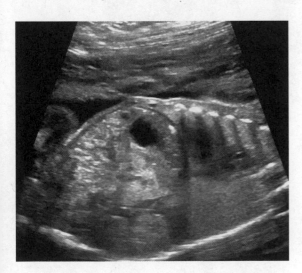

1. Describe the anatomy in this fetal abdomen and relate the significance to FGR.

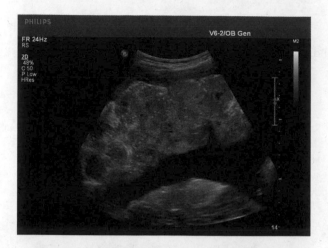

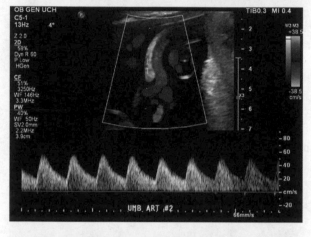

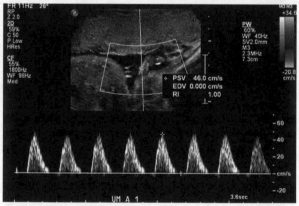

A

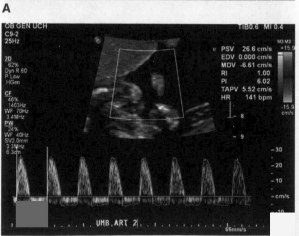

B

2. Describe the placenta.

3. Explain the fetal anatomy under interrogation. Is the waveform normal or abnormal for this vessel?

4. Discuss image A and B waveforms regarding the fetal umbilical artery.

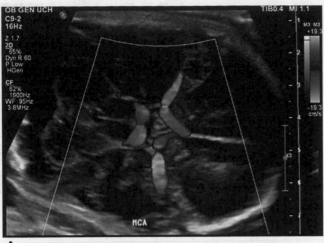

A

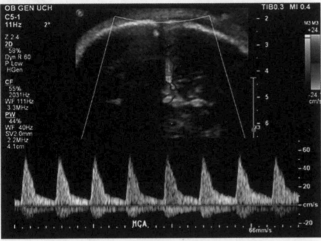

B

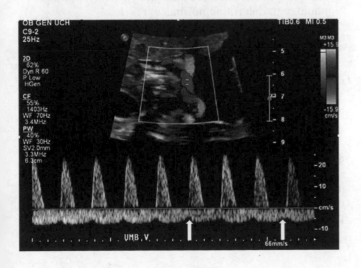

5. Describe the fetal anatomy. What is color Doppler demonstrating in image A? State the type of waveform seen in image B.

6. Explain the spectral Doppler tracing of the umbilical cord in an FGR fetus.

CHAPTER 33

Patterns of Fetal Anomalies

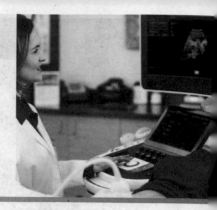

REVIEW OF GLOSSARY TERMS

Matching

Match the key terms with their definitions.

KEY TERMS

1. _____ triple screen

2. _____ multifactorial

3. _____ analyte

4. _____ karyotype

5. _____ meiosis

6. _____ quadruple screen

7. _____ Inhibin A

8. _____ mitosis

9. _____ human chorionic gonadotropin (hCG)

10. _____ pregnancy-associated plasma protein A (PAPP-A)

11. _____ alpha-fetoprotein (AFP)

12. _____ preeclampsia

13. _____ aneuploidy

14. _____ mosaicism

15. _____ unconjugated estriol (uE3)

16. _____ haploid

DEFINITIONS

a. Serum protein produced by the fetal yolk sac and liver that aids in the detection of neural tube defects, ventral wall defects, skin disorders, and in rare cases, nephrosis

b. Any substance measured in a laboratory such as AFP, inhibin A, or human chorionic gonadotropin

c. Abnormal number of chromosomes

d. Normal number of chromosomes in a cell

e. Testing for maternal levels of AFP, unconjugated estriol, hCG, and inhibin A

f. Hormone secreted by immature placenta

g. Protein secreted by the corpus luteum and placenta

h. Arrangement of chromosomes by type, size, and morphology to determine normalcy

i. Presence of two different types of cell genotypes (karyotype) in an individual

j. Division of a cell resulting in the normal haploid number

k. Division of a cell resulting in which there is a reduction, by half, in the normal haploid number of chromosomes

l. Triad of hypertension, fluid retention (edema), and proteinuria occurring after 20 weeks' gestation

m. Placental syncytiotrophoblastic hormone found in the maternal bloodstream

n. Involving several different factors

o. Testing for maternal levels of AFP, uE3, and hCG

p. Hormone produced by the syncytiotrophoblast

ANATOMY AND PHYSIOLOGY REVIEW

Image Labeling

Complete the labels in the images that follow.

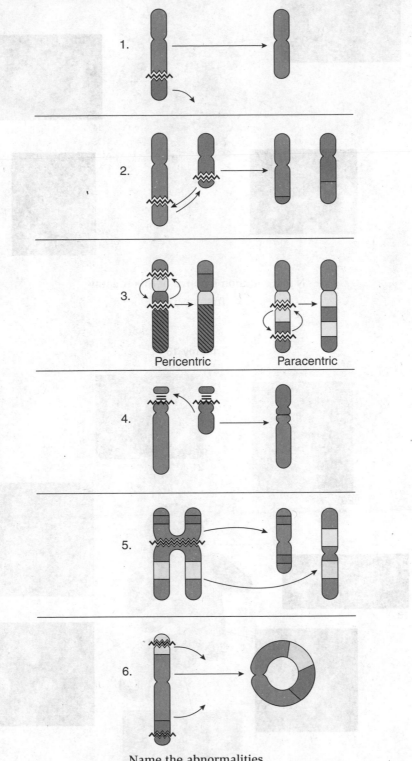

1.

2.

3. Pericentric   Paracentric

4.

5.

6.

Name the abnormalities.

Human chromosome structural abnormalities

Trisomy 13

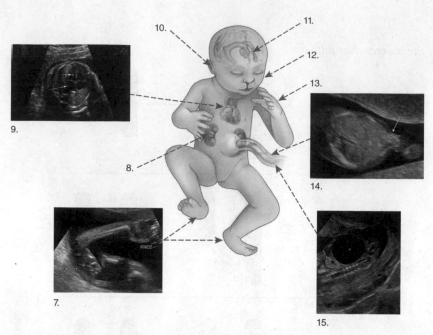

Name common features of this trisomy.

Trisomy 13

Trisomy 18

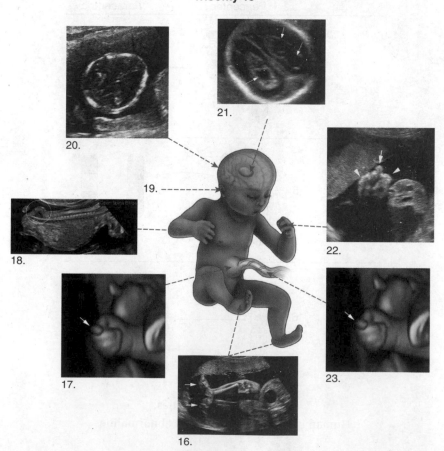

Name common features of this trisomy.

Trisomy 18

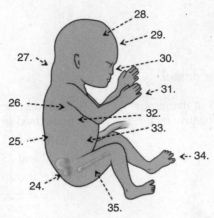

Name common features of this trisomy.

Trisomy 21

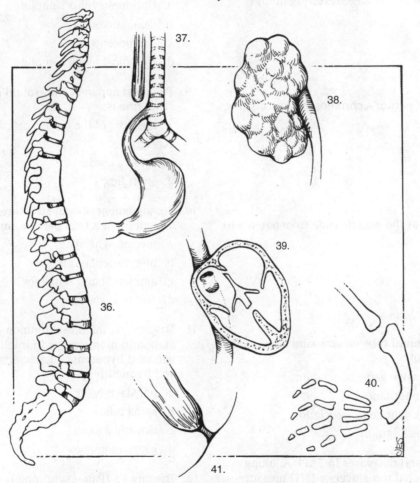

Name features of this anomaly.

VACTERL association

CHAPTER REVIEW

Multiple Choice

Complete each question by circling the best answer.

1. A pattern of multiple anomalies seen in numerous individuals not related to a single causative factor or pathology is a(n):
   a. syndrome
   b. disruption
   c. malformation
   d. association

2. Structural abnormalities in the chromosomes are most often a result of breakage resulting from:
   a. deletion
   b. inversion
   c. chemical agents
   d. translocation

3. The definition of a part of a chromosome rearranging within itself is:
   a. inversion
   b. insertion
   c. deletion
   d. translocation

4. The transmission of the genetic code from parents to offspring is:
   a. association
   b. insertion
   c. inheritance
   d. sequence

5. Cardiac defects, neural tube defects, and facial clefting are examples of:
   a. autosomal recessive gene association
   b. multifactorial inheritance
   c. autosomal dominant gene association
   d. X-linked gene association

6. Increases in hCG and decreases in PAPP-A, along with increased nuchal translucency (NT) measurements, have been associated with:
   a. Trisomy 13
   b. Trisomy 18
   c. Trisomy 21
   d. VACTERL association

7. Second-semester biochemical screening should be performed between:
   a. 10 and 13 weeks
   b. 20 and 25 weeks
   c. 18 and 26 weeks
   d. 15 and 20 weeks

8. Select the choice that is not associated with diagnosing aneuploidy.
   a. Chorionic villus sampling
   b. Qualitative hCG
   c. Amniocentesis
   d. Umbilical blood sampling

9. The most apparent ultrasound finding with Aicardi syndrome is:
   a. agenesis of the corpus callosum
   b. club feet
   c. ectopic cordis
   d. short limbs

10. Entanglement of fetal structures or the obvious disruption of a fetal part by amniotic sheets is:
    a. uterine synechiae
    b. uterine septations
    c. amniotic band sequence
    d. amniotic sheets

11. Trisomy 21, the most common pattern of malformation in man, results in intellectual disabilities, neonatal hypotonia, characteristic facial deformities, and frequently:
    a. polydactyly
    b. spina bifida
    c. cloverleaf skull
    d. heart anomalies

12. Trisomy 13 (Patau syndrome):
    a. is frequently related to advanced maternal age
    b. demonstrates no cranial anomalies
    c. includes a short umbilical cord
    d. involves the vertebrae with severe kyphoscoliosis

13. An anomaly, either single or multiple, in which the structure or tissue is abnormal from the beginning, such as clefting of the lip, is a(n):
    a. association
    b. malformation
    c. sequence
    d. deformation

14. The five findings—macroglossia, anterior wall defects, hypoglycemia at birth, macrosomia, and hemi-hyperplasia—suggest a diagnosis of:
    a. HOS syndrome
    b. Trisomy 13
    c. Cri-du-chat syndrome
    d. Beckwith-Wiedemann syndrome

15. VACTERL syndrome:
    a. is a collection of fetal anomalies
    b. is best diagnosed with inhibin A
    c. is determined with amniocentesis
    d. requires multiple anomalies including hip dysplasia

16. The characteristics of renal dysplasia, limb anomalies, and encephalocele describe the rare syndrome:
    a. Goldenhar
    b. Trisomy 13
    c. Meckel-Gruber
    d. Monosomy X

17. Turner syndrome relates to:
    a. oligohydramnios owing to inadequate urine production
    b. the absence of a sex chromosome
    c. limb amputation
    d. hand anomalies

18. An anomaly in which the structure of tissue lacks the normal organization of cells is a(n):
    a. syndrome
    b. disruption
    c. dysplasia
    d. association

19. A syndrome that is separated into two subgroups with one having craniofacial defects and one having a short cord, anal atresia, lumbosacral meningocele, and urogenital malformations is:
    a. Patua syndrome
    b. Cri-du-chat syndrome
    c. Beckwith-Wiedemann syndrome
    d. limb–body wall complex

20. A condition that provides no known lab values and is known as the cardiac–limb syndrome is:
    a. Holt-Oran syndrome
    b. CHARGE syndrome
    c. caudal dysplasia sequence
    d. Wilms syndrome

Fill-in-the-Blank

1. Turner syndrome is known as _____ and only affects the _____ gender.

2. Turner syndrome results from the absence of one of the two _____ chromosomes.

3. Trisomy 13 is also known as _____, Trisomy 21 is known as _____, and Trisomy 18 is known as _____.

4. Having one extra chromosome in a set or missing a chromosome from a set are examples of _____.

5. In a Trisomy 21 fetus, a first-trimester ultrasound examination often displays a missing _____ bone.

6. Two environmental teratogens that mimic genetic defects are _____ and _____.

7. A well-known and reliable screening test that evaluates the risk to the general population for aneuploidy is _____.

8. _____ is the main characteristic of Apert syndrome that results in changes of head and face shape.

9. Trisomy 18 is also known as _____ and occurs mostly in the _____ gender.

10. Defects of the sacrum, lumbar vertebrae, and sacral agenesis are anomalies related to _____. Extreme temperature, x-rays, and lithium are known to induce this malformation.

11. Also known as cardiac–limb syndrome, _____ is characterized by anomalies of the upper limbs and the heart.

12. The classic sonographic finding of Turner syndrome is a _____.

13. A fetus that demonstrates hypertelorism, downward slanting eyes, and posteriorly rotated and low-set ears, has _____ syndrome. The short stature, neck webbing, and cardiac anomalies compare to Turner syndrome.

14. The presence of a complete extra set of chromosomes is called _____.

15. _____ band sequence, or _____ band syndrome, begins with the rupture of the amnion and subsequently results in the entrapment of fetal parts.

16. When a mother carries a gene that expresses itself in a male child, this is considered an _____-linked chromosome.

17. A pattern of the anomalies colobomatous malformation, heart defects, atresia choanae, retardation (mental and growth deficiencies), genital hypoplasia, and ear anomalies equates to _____ syndrome.

18. Cystic hygroma is common to Turner syndrome and Noonan syndrome; however, the identification of a _____ genitalia differentiates Noonan syndrome from Turner syndrome.

19. Agenesis of the corpus callosum, dysgenesis of the corpus callosum, cortical malformations, brain asymmetry, microcephaly, choroid plexus cysts, porencephalic cysts, choroid plexus papilloma, Dandy-Walker malformation, and brain calcifications indicate _____ syndrome.

20. Most triploidy pregnancies are owing to two _____ one egg or from an extra chromosome set from the mother.

Short Answer

1. Discuss risk factors related to chromosomal abnormalities.

2. List the four biochemical markers that are essential to modern prenatal care. What is the alternative name for this screening test?

3. Compare and contrast autosomal dominant with autosomal recessive genetic coding. List the syndromes, sequences, and associations related to autosomal dominant coding.

4. What syndromes affect fetal kidneys and genital system?

IMAGE EVALUATION/PATHOLOGY

Review the images and answer the following questions.

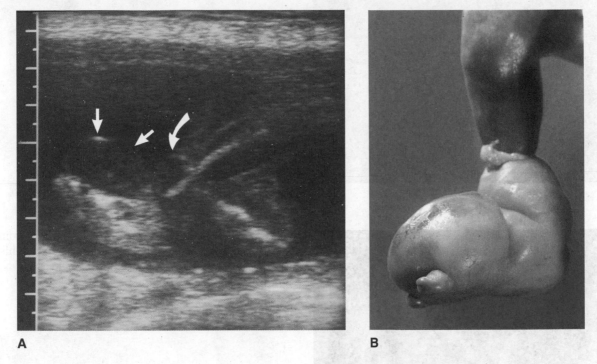

1. Explain the images of the same prenatal and postnatal fetal foot. Offer a diagnosis.

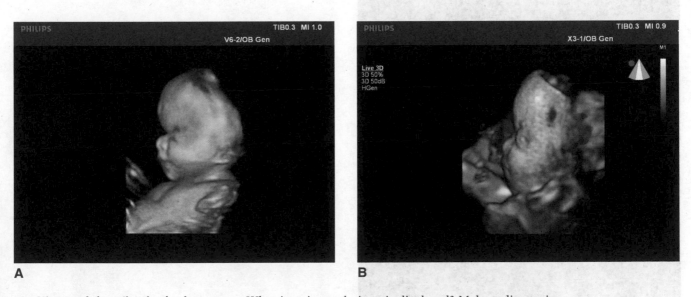

2. View and describe the fetal anatomy. What imaging technique is displayed? Make a diagnosis.

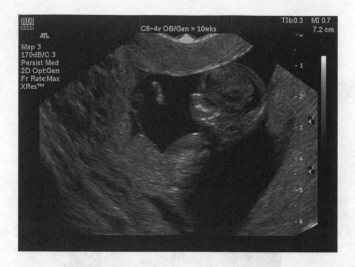

3. Explain the image, make a diagnosis, and explain possible related findings for the anomaly.

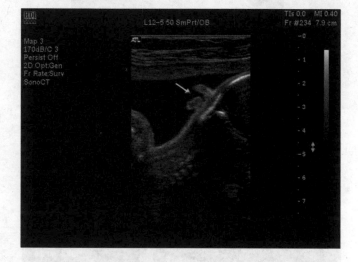

4. Describe the abnormal structure. What syndromes in this chapter suggested syndromes related to this fetal structure?

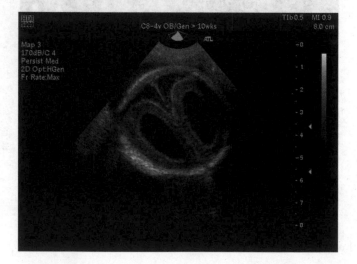

5. Name the anatomy. Offer a diagnosis.

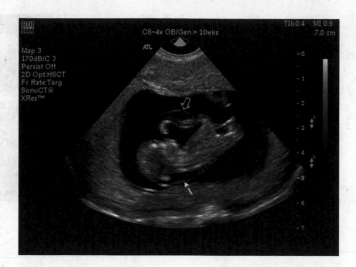

6. Explain what the posterior solid arrow is pointing to. Also, what is the anterior open arrow directed at?

CHAPTER 34

Effects of Maternal Disease on Pregnancy

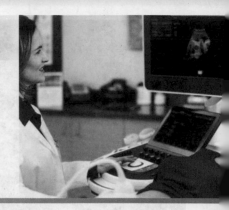

REVIEW OF GLOSSARY TERMS

Matching

Match the key terms with their definitions.

KEY TERMS

1. _____ systemic lupus erythematous

2. _____ hyperthyroidism

3. _____ pinocytosis

4. _____ TORCH

5. _____ thrombophilias

6. _____ nonimmune hydrops

7. _____ cytomegalovirus (CMV)

8. _____ hypothyroidism

9. _____ varicella-zoster infection

10. _____ thalassemia

11. _____ diabetes mellitus

12. _____ hyperparathyroidism

13. _____ germ line

14. _____ eclampsia

15. _____ gestational diabetes

16. _____ Rh isoimmunization

17. _____ rubella (aka German measles)

18. _____ phenylketonuria

19. _____ human immunodeficiency virus (HIV)

DEFINITIONS

a. Overactive thyroid gland; pathologically excessive production of thyroid hormones or the condition resulting from excessive production of thyroid hormones

b. Underactive thyroid gland; a glandular disorder resulting from insufficient production of thyroid hormones

c. Excessive secretion of parathyroid hormone resulting in abnormally high levels of calcium in the blood; can affect many systems of the body (especially causing bone resorption and osteoporosis)

d. Genetic disorder of metabolism; lack of the enzyme needed to turn phenylalanine into tyrosine, which results in an accumulation of phenylalanine in the body fluids, which causes various degrees of mental deficiency

e. A mechanism by which cells ingest extracellular fluid contents

f. Development of immunities to Rh-positive blood antigens from a fetus by an RH-negative woman

g. Accumulation of fluid in fetal tissues in the form of ascites, pleural fluid, and skin edema resulting from factors other than a fetomaternal blood group incompatibility

h. Congenital form of anemia occurring mostly in blacks; characterized by crescent-shaped blood cells

i. Inherited form of anemia caused by faulty synthesis of hemoglobin

j. Abnormal condition of pregnancy characterized by hypertension, edema, and protein in the urine

k. Coma and seizures in second and third trimesters following preeclampsia

l. Maternal high blood pressure that was diagnosed prior to pregnancy

m. Thrombophilia or hypercoagulability is the propensity to develop thrombosis (blood clots) because of a coagulation abnormality.

20. _____ toxemia (aka preeclampsia)

21. _____ parvovirus B19

22. _____ sickle cell anemia

23. _____ Epstein-Barr virus

24. _____ coronavirus (COVID-19)

25. _____ essential hypertension

26. _____ toxoplasmosis

27. _____ intrauterine growth restriction (IUGR)

28. _____ influenza

29. _____ Zika virus

n. Inflammatory disease of connective tissue with variable features including fever, weakness, fatigability, joint pains, and skin lesions on the face, neck, or arms

o. Estimated fetal weight <10th percentile for the gestational age

p. Chickenpox infection

q. Herpes virus that causes infectious mononucleosis

r. Ovum or sperm (germ cells) that have genetic material that passes to offspring

s. Acute febrile highly contagious viral disease

t. Human immunodeficiency virus that progresses into AIDS (acquired immune deficiency syndrome)

u. Parasitic infection transmitted to humans from undercooked meat or contact with cat feces

v. Includes toxoplasmosis, other viruses (syphilis, varicella-zoster, parvovirus B19), rubella, cytomegalovirus, and herpes infections

w. Contagious viral disease that is a milder form of measles lasting 3 or 4 days

x. Condition in which women without previously diagnosed diabetes exhibit high blood glucose levels during pregnancy

y. Any of a group of herpes viruses that enlarge epithelial cells and can cause birth defects; can affect humans with impaired immunologic systems

z. Erythema infectiosum or fifth disease; spreading via the upper respiratory tract, this virus affects children more strongly than adults

aa. Mosquito-borne single-stranded RNA virus related to the dengue virus

bb. An infectious disease caused by a newly discovered coronavirus

cc. Diabetes caused by a relative or absolute deficiency of insulin and characterized by polyuria

ANATOMY AND PHYSIOLOGY REVIEW

Image Labeling

Complete the labels in the images that follow.

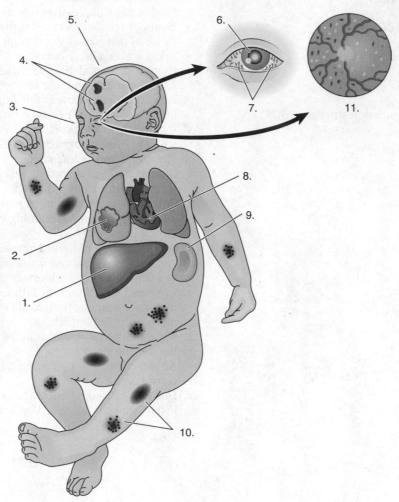

TORCH infections

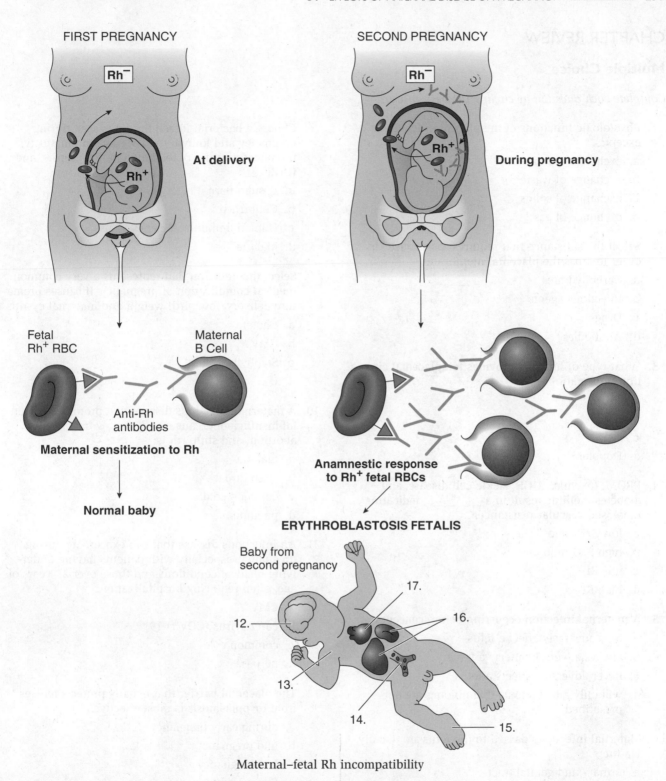

FIRST PREGNANCY

Rh⁻

At delivery

Rh⁺

SECOND PREGNANCY

Rh⁻

During pregnancy

Rh⁺

Fetal
Rh⁺ RBC

Maternal
B Cell

Anti-Rh
antibodies

Maternal sensitization to Rh

Normal baby

**Anamnestic response
to Rh⁺ fetal RBCs**

ERYTHROBLASTOSIS FETALIS

Baby from
second pregnancy

12.

13.

14.

17.

16.

15.

Maternal–fetal Rh incompatibility

CHAPTER REVIEW

Multiple Choice

Complete each question by circling the best answer.

1. Physiologic functions of the placenta include all except:
   a. exchange of nutrients
   b. exchange of waste
   c. exchange of solids
   d. exchange of gas

2. Select the substance that requires "assistance" in order to cross the placental membrane.
   a. Carbohydrates
   b. Infectious agents
   c. Drugs
   d. Antibodies

3. What type of imaging provides fetoplacental circulation information?
   a. TV
   b. EV
   c. TA
   d. Doppler

4. PROM, toxemia, IUGR, sickle cell disease, and diabetes mellitus result in a _____ indicating increased vascular resistance.
   a. low S/D ratio
   b. high S/D ratio
   c. low RI
   d. high RI

5. A maternal infection occurring before conception:
   a. may adversely affect a fetus
   b. always adversely affects a fetus
   c. never adversely affects a fetus
   d. will only affect a fetus if antibiotics are not prescribed

6. Maternal infections passed to the fetus are usually via the:
   a. urinary and genital tract
   b. circulatory and respiratory systems
   c. genital tract and circulatory systems
   d. urinary and respiratory systems

7. A rare viral infection that is linked to stillbirth, low infant birth weight, congenital heart anomalies, and microphthalmia is:
   a. HIV
   b. IUGR
   c. EBV
   d. varicella-zoster

8. Choose a bacterial infection that is seen during pregnancy and known to cause fetal prematurity, prolonged rupture of fetal membranes, sepsis, and IUGR.
   a. Epstein-Barr
   b. Gonorrhea
   c. Human immunodeficiency virus
   d. Malaria

9. Select the infection that represents a very common medical complication of pregnancy. It causes premature delivery/low birth weight and maternal cystitis.
   a. Cholera
   b. CMV
   c. Staphylococcus
   d. UTI

10. A maternal infectious disease that promotes placental insufficiency, causing IUGR, low birth weight, abortion, and stillbirth is:
   a. malaria
   b. strep throat
   c. common cold
   d. pneumonia

11. An infectious disease that can exacerbate during pregnancy, especially with patients having underlying medical conditions and those over 25 years of age, often requiring hospitalization:
   a. CMV
   b. coronavirus (COVID-19)
   c. common cold
   d. herpes

12. The placental barrier that usually protects fetuses from toxoplasmosis is most effective:
   a. during early pregnancy
   b. mid pregnancy
   c. late pregnancy
   d. throughout the entire pregnancy

13. Fetal malformations occurring in the first trimester which consist of cataracts, cardiac defects, and deafness are caused by:
   a. mumps
   b. 3-day measles
   c. herpes virus
   d. pertussis

14. Periventricular echogenic calcifications visualized in the fetal cranium are commonly related to:
    a. hyperthyroidism and parathyroidism
    b. Rh isoimmunization
    c. chickenpox
    d. rubella and parvovirus B19

15. Select the type of diabetes that occurs only during pregnancy and affects about 7% of all pregnant women.
    a. Type I
    b. Type II
    c. Monogenic
    d. Gestational

16. A glucose tolerance test:
    a. is usually performed between weeks 24 and 28
    b. checks the glucose level 2 hours after p.o. ingestion of a glucose solution
    c. that displays a 1-hour elevated level will require a 4-hour tolerance test
    d. is requested only if there is a family history of diabetes mellitus

17. Isoimmunized pregnancies can result in all except:
    a. erythroblastosis fetalis
    b. hepatosplenomegaly
    c. immune hydrops fetalis
    d. Rh factor

18. Maternal edema, hypertension, proteinuria, and nervous system irritability define:
    a. thrombophilia symptoms
    b. toxemia/hypertension symptoms
    c. maternal rubella symptoms
    d. maternal viral infection symptoms

19. The safest time for a female diagnosed with systemic lupus erythematosus to produce a pregnancy is:
    a. early in the childbearing years
    b. when disease activity is controlled by small doses of steroids and aspirin
    c. after multiple treatments of clomiphene
    d. following blood transfusion

20. Select the maternal disease that is least likely to affect a fetus's heart:
    a. Influenza
    b. TORCH
    c. Thalassemia
    d. EBV

Fill-in-the-Blank

1. The _____ plays a role as a barrier in preventing or facilitating the transmission of maternal disease to the fetus.

2. Substances and agents that move across the placental barrier, harming the developing fetus are _____, _____, and antibodies.

3. Maternal hypertension _____ uteroplacental blood flow.

4. Normally, as pregnancy progresses, diastolic flow _____, representing _____ resistance to flow.

5. Toxemia (preeclampsia) of pregnancy is a _____-trimester disease characterized by maternal edema, hypertension, proteinuria, and central nervous system irritability.

6. Of the patients diagnosed with preeclampsia, 2% to 12% are affected by the _____ syndrome.

7. Patients with UTIs during pregnancy should be treated with _____ and monitored by frequent urine _____.

8. Maternal malaria promotes placental _____, causing IUGR, low birth weight, abortion, and stillbirth.

9. Fetal _____, a diagnostic test, helps detect heart abnormalities in patients exposed to CMV and rubella.

10. If severe toxoplasmosis infection occurs, the outcome presents as central nervous system anomalies such as _____, _____, _____, _____, and mental retardation.

11. Cyanotic heart disease results in premature birth, IUGR, and miscarriages, possibly owing to the lower _____ content in maternal circulation.

12. If an obstetric patient is infected with parvovirus B19, ultrasound to image anatomy and measurement of the _____ of the middle cerebral artery are noninvasive procedures to diagnose fetal anemia and nonimmune hydrops.

13. Cesarean section delivery is indicated in the event of _____ virus in the maternal genital tract.

14. Congenital malformations seen with diabetes are related to high blood sugar levels resulting in disruption of embryonic _____.

15. The preferred predictor of neonatal weight in the third trimester is the _____ measurement.

16. Hyperthyroidism produces thyroxine that causes a significant increase of _____-birth weight infants.

17. Phenylketonuria (PKU) control is by following a low-_____, low-protein _____.

18. Rh isoimmunization refers to the development of maternal _____ to the surface antigens on fetal _____ blood cells.

19. Rigid irregularly shaped blood cells that occur mostly in African Americans in the United States is a cause of _____.

20. Ingestion of raw meat, contaminated water, and contact with feline feces is advised against for the obstetrical patient owing to the risk of acquiring _____.

Short Answer

1. Define TORCH.

2. Explain possible fetal outcomes with a woman who shows serologic evidence of previous varicella-zoster.

3. A primigravida 24-year-old diabetic has concerns about her endocrine/metabolic disorder in regard to her unborn child. Explain congenital anomalies frequently noted in infants of diabetic mothers and how to decrease the incidence of congenital anomalies.

4. A large city hospital was reported to have an abnormally high level of babies born to mothers known to consume and abuse alcohol during pregnancy. List findings that ultrasound may discover prior to delivery regarding these fetuses.

IMAGE EVALUATION/PATHOLOGY

Review the images and answer the following questions.

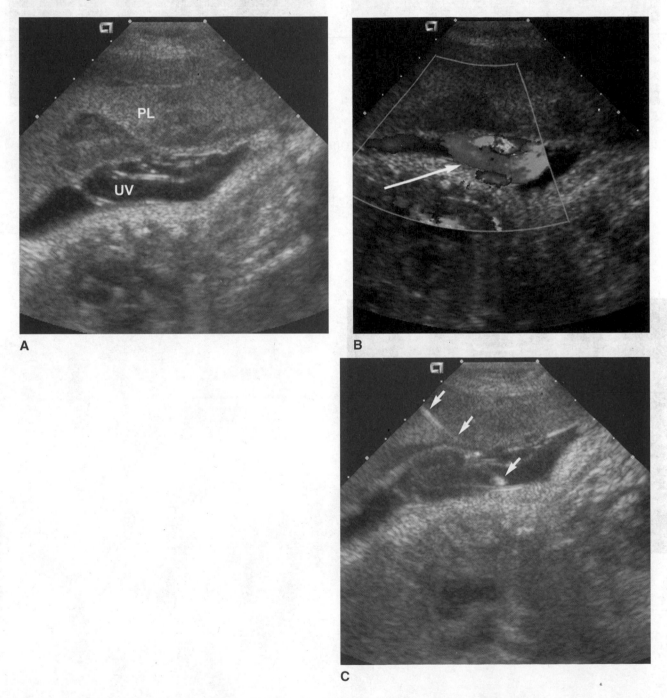

A

B

C

1. Review the images and explain the invasive ultrasound procedure that is documented. See arrows in image C.

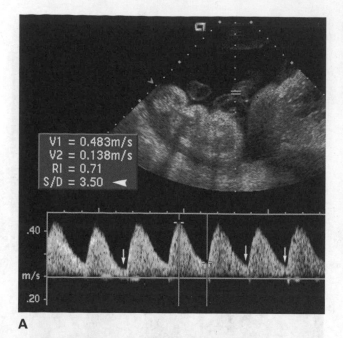

A

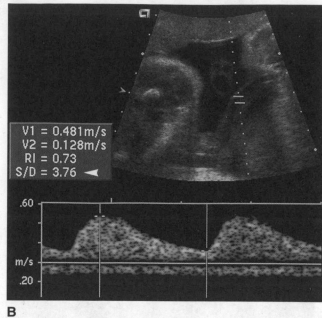

B

2. In images A and B, spectral Doppler was performed. Offer a diagnosis.

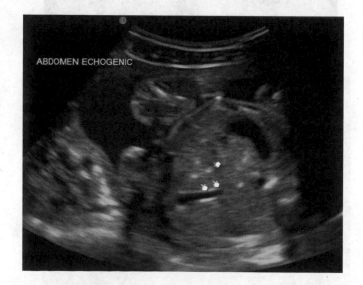

3. Explain the foci within a fetal liver. Name a likely diagnosis.

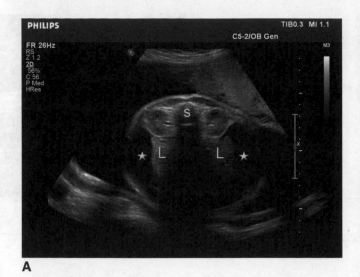

A

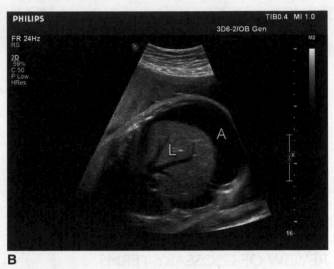

B

4. Describe the findings that are demonstrated in the chest image (A) and abdominal image (B) of this fetus diagnosed with hydrops fetalis. What irregularities may be noted in the fetal cranium and neck with this condition?

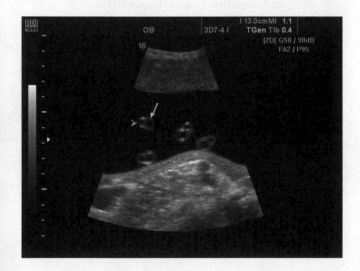

5. Name the anatomy.

CHAPTER 35

The Postpartum Uterus

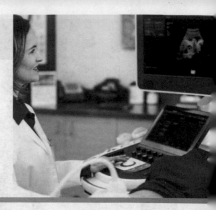

REVIEW OF GLOSSARY TERMS

Matching

Match the key terms with their definitions.

KEY TERMS

1. _____ hysterectomy

2. _____ decidua basalis

3. _____ atony

4. _____ nephrolithiasis

5. _____ involution

6. _____ coagulopathy

7. _____ venogram

8. _____ emboli

9. _____ thrombophlebitis

10. _____ chorioamnionitis

11. _____ hematoma

12. _____ intravenous pyelogram (IVP)

DEFINITIONS

a. Radiographic examination of the vein performed after injection of a radiopaque contrast medium
b. Formation of a blood clot owing to inflammation
c. Stones within the kidney
d. Radiographic images of the kidneys, ureters, and bladder after injection of a radiopaque dye
e. Reduction of an organ to its normal size and appearance
f. Removal of the uterus
g. Collection of blood outside the vessels
h. Moving particles, such as thrombosis or air, within the bloodstream
i. Portion of the uterine lining which forms the maternal portion of the placenta
j. Defect in the body's clotting mechanism resulting in bleeding
k. Inflammation of the amnion and chorion owing to a bacterial infection
l. Lack of normal muscle tone

CHAPTER REVIEW

Multiple Choice

Complete each question by circling the best answer.

1. The puerperium:
   a. describes the postdelivery condition of the female external genitalia
   b. starts immediately post delivery including the placenta and continues until the uterus retains its prenatal shape
   c. is an infection of the placental site within the uterus
   d. extends from placental delivery until the first normal menstruation

2. Lactation termination usually produces:
   a. anovulation
   b. menstrual resumption
   c. breast lumps
   d. excessive quantities of breast milk

3. Sonography in the puerperium period is used for all except:
   a. evaluating puerperal infection
   b. postpartum hemorrhage
   c. complications following cesarean delivery
   d. to routinely determine whether the uterus has returned to prepregnancy state

4. Select the true statement regarding the postpartum uterus.
   a. The internal os will be visualized as closed and well delineated following placental delivery.
   b. The endometrium will measure 3 to 8 mm within 24 hours of delivery.
   c. Free fluid in the endometrial cavity indicates intrauterine infection.
   d. Longitudinal uterine measurements range from 14 to 25 cm.

5. During pregnancy, ovaries generally:
   a. remain the same as prepregnancy state with the exception of a few more cysts in the first trimester
   b. involute
   c. enlarge owing to hormone production
   d. develop a thickened outer cortex

6. A placenta that completely invades the uterine myometrium extending into the serosa is:
   a. placenta abruption
   b. placenta percreta
   c. placenta accreta
   d. placenta increta

7. Select the condition that is not likely to be related to postpartum hemorrhage.
   a. Decreased hematocrit
   b. Shock
   c. Hypertension
   d. Hysterectomy

8. RPOC has a similar sonographic appearance to:
   a. highly echogenic mass in the endometrial canal
   b. increta
   c. a placental polyp with positive blood flow
   d. a hemorrhagic cystic collection

9. Usually the first indication of uterine (puerperium) infection is:
   a. excessive vaginal bleeding
   b. flank pain
   c. uterine "afterpains"
   d. uterine tenderness

10. The only infection that is not typically related to postpartum infection is:
    a. UTI
    b. salpingitis
    c. thrombophlebitis
    d. breast infection

11. Which of the following is not identified with uterine atony?
    a. Chorioamnionitis
    b. Prolonged labor
    c. Oligohydramnios
    d. Macrosomy

12. The most common signs of POVT are:
    a. fever, right-sided pelvic mass, and pelvic pain
    b. nausea and groin pain
    c. vomiting and flank pain
    d. bowel ileus and hypertension

13. Cesarean section delivery:
    a. has an increased risk of infection
    b. is mostly performed with a vertical incision
    c. requires a low-frequency transducer when hematoma occurs adjacent to the bladder flap
    d. accounts for approximately 13.8% of all U.S. deliveries

14. The most frequent site of postpartum thrombophlebitis is:
    a. left ovarian vein
    b. fundal uterine vein
    c. deep cervical vein
    d. right ovarian vein

15. Endometritis:
    a. is an infection of the endometrium that may extend to the myometrium, which may lead to postpartum bleeding
    b. appears as an extremely thin endometrium and irregular walls
    c. produces a fluid-filled endometrium
    d. causes a flaccid uterus post delivery

Fill-in-the-Blank

1. The postpartum period may also be called the _____.

2. Complications seen most frequently following cesarean section are _____ and _____ at the incision site.

3. It is essential to remember to use a _____ pressure than when imaging the nongravid uterus.

4. If a post C-section patient cannot tolerate transabdominal or transvaginal imaging, the _____ or _____ imaging method may visualize the C-section incision.

5. The adnexal ligaments of the postpartum patient are typically _____ immediately following delivery, usually returning to their pregravid states within _____.

6. Postpartum hemorrhage is considered over _____ mL of blood with a vaginal delivery and over _____ mL of blood in a cesarean delivery.

7. The cause of placenta accreta, percreta, and increta is complete or partial absence of the _____.

8. Antepartum rupture of the uterus causes emergency delivery and _____.

9. Sonography helps identify the multiple intraplacental _____ that are indicators of placental invasion of the myometrium.

10. The sonographic appearance of endometritis is that of a _____, irregular endometrium that may have _____ in the endocervical canal.

11. Retained products of conception image as a _____ mass within an irregularly shaped uterus.

12. Sonographically, POVT images as a dilated anechoic to hypoechoic _____ structure extending superiorly from the adnexa.

13. Hematomas found in the bladder flap region are sonographically _____ with ill-defined borders that range in size from less than 1 cm to greater than 15 cm.

14. A _____-frequency transducer is sometimes needed to adequately assess postpartum cesarean section hematomas.

15. Infections following cesarean sections have appearances of anechoic, _____, _____, and with or without definite margins.

Short Answer

1. Offer an explanation for the uterus acquiring infection in the postpartum state.

2. Define RPOC and describe the sonographic appearance.

3. Explain complications involved with a cesarean section incision.

IMAGE EVALUATION/PATHOLOGY

Review the images and answer the following questions.

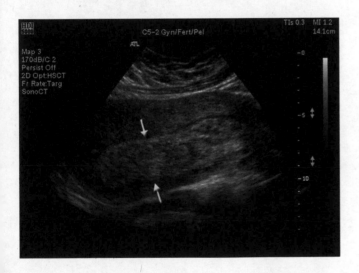

1. Describe the finding in the postpartum uterus (arrows). What factors should be considered when assessing this patient? Recommend a treatment plan, if any.

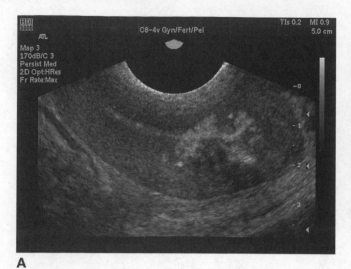

A

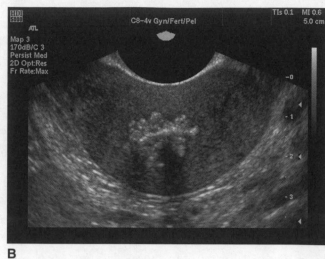

B

2. Diagnose the sagittal and transverse views of the transvaginal uterine images.

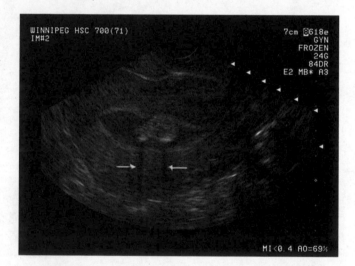

3. Diagnose the image. This is an image of a uterus after an elective termination was performed.

4. Describe the hematoma.

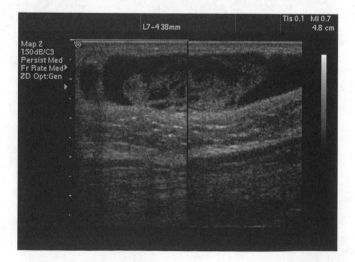

PART FOUR

ADVANCED IMAGING

CHAPTER 36

Interventional Ultrasound

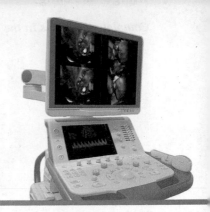

REVIEW OF GLOSSARY TERMS

Matching

Match the key terms with their definitions.

KEY TERMS

1. _____ coelocentesis

2. _____ petri dish

3. _____ amniocentesis

4. _____ transcervical

5. _____ multifetal

6. _____ advanced maternal age (AMA)

7. _____ culdocentesis

8. _____ abscess drainage

9. _____ biopsy

10. _____ oocyte retrieval

11. _____ endovaginal ultrasound

12. _____ chorionic villus sampling (CVS)

13. _____ percutaneous umbilical blood sampling (PUBS, aka cordocentesis)

DEFINITIONS

a. Woman 35 years of age or older
b. Sampling of fetal blood via the umbilical cord
c. Through the cervix
d. Removal of the infected fluid
e. Round dish used to culture fetal tissue or cells
f. Sampling of chorionic villus of the placenta
g. Early sampling of the exocoelomic cavity fluid via placenta-free areas
h. Procedure in which oocytes are aspirated from the ovaries
i. Aspiration of peritoneal fluid from the posterior cul-de-sac
j. Noninvasive ultrasound examination performed with a transducer inserted into the vagina
k. Sampling of amniotic fluid
l. Procedure to remove a piece of tissue or a sample of cells
m. More than one fetus

ANATOMY AND PHYSIOLOGY REVIEW

Image Labeling

Complete the labels in the images that follow.

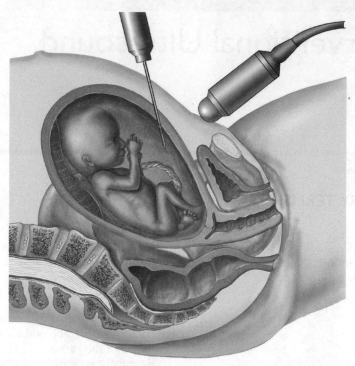

Pregnancy sampling—name the procedure.

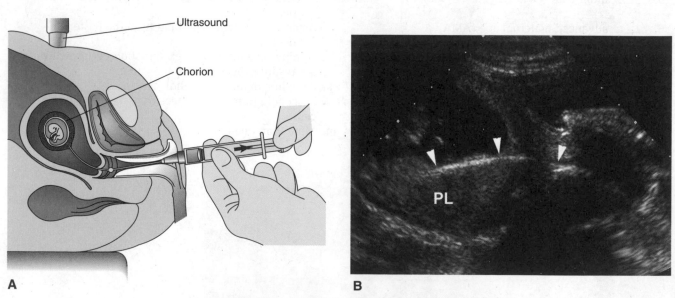

Target area for sampling—name the procedure.

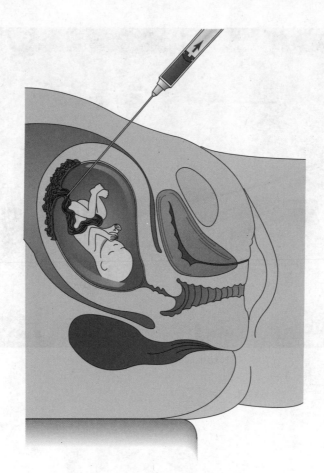

Sampling—name the procedure.

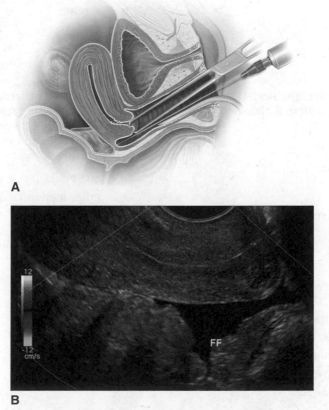

Fluid extraction—name the procedure

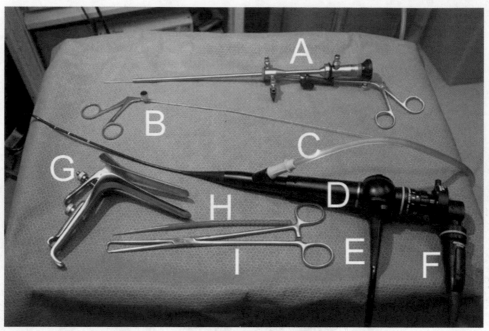

Hysteroscopy equipment

CHAPTER REVIEW

Multiple Choice

Complete each question by circling the best answer.

1. A common clinical technique for retrieving living fetal cells/cell products from the pregnant uterus is:
   a. PUBS
   b. amniotic villus sampling
   c. amniocentesis
   d. culdocentesis

2. An ultrasound procedure that obtains fetal blood via a needle inserted into the maternal abdomen is:
   a. fetal transfusion
   b. reduction
   c. fetal rapid blood culture
   d. PUBS

3. Amniocentesis testing is recommended at:
   a. 6 to 8 weeks
   b. 8 to 14 weeks
   c. 14 to 20 weeks
   d. 20 to 30 weeks

4. Fetal blood sampling occurs at the:
   a. venous cord insertion site
   b. arterial cord insertion site
   c. intrahepatic umbilical vein
   d. intrahepatic umbilical artery

5. Vaginal coelocentesis can provide a sample of extra-amniotic fluid as early as:
   a. 8 weeks
   b. 12 weeks
   c. 10 weeks
   d. 6 weeks

6. Women whose maternal serum alpha-fetoprotein (MSAFP) screening results reveal a value below the mean levels for a given gestational age have been associated with an increased risk for:
   a. trisomy
   b. spina bifida
   c. cardiac malformations
   d. anencephaly

7. Indications for using an endovaginal transducer are all except:
   a. ovarian cyst aspiration
   b. embryo transfer
   c. hemoglobinopathies
   d. IUCD position

8. The main purpose of multifetal pregnancy reduction is to:
   a. limit the number of children a couple chooses to produce
   b. reduce the number of embryos to improve survival for the remaining ones
   c. decrease physician liability in a multiple pregnancy
   d. decrease the financial burden of multiples

9. Hysterosonosalpingography should always be performed during the _____ of the menstrual cycle.
   a. early follicular phase
   b. late proliferative phase
   c. secretory phase
   d. menstrual phase

10. Select the most common endovaginal ultrasound puncture procedure.
    a. Percutaneous pelvic mass biopsy
    b. Embryo transfer
    c. Radiotherapy planning and monitoring
    d. Oocyte retrieval

11. Culdocentesis is performed to:
    a. collect a sampling of the exocoelomic cavity fluid
    b. acquire fluid posterior to the lower uterus
    c. place a pelvic drainage catheter
    d. diagnose inflammatory intestinal wall

12. Ultrasound is used to guide local treatment of the drug _____ for ectopic pregnancy resolution.
    a. methotrexate
    b. reprotox
    c. methohexital
    d. repronex

13. Which imaging modality is most useful in diagnosing ectopic pregnancy?
    a. Spectral Doppler ultrasound
    b. MRI with contrast
    c. Color Doppler ultrasound
    d. TCD

14. The gold standard procedure for establishing tubal condition is:
    a. sonohysterosalpingography
    b. laparoscopy
    c. HSG
    d. hysteroscopy

15. 3D endovaginal sonography is useful in the detection of all except:
    a. IUCD position
    b. IUCD shaft and branch orientation
    c. detection of IUCD
    d. IUCD hormone level

16. Choose a disadvantage of CVS.
    a. Accuracy
    b. Early genetic diagnosis
    c. False-positive result
    d. Ability to obtain living fetal cells or products of them

17. The legal limit for elective termination of pregnancy in the United States is determined by:
    a. county guidelines
    b. state laws
    c. findings/laboratory results and fetal gestational age
    d. health and welfare of the pregnant woman

18. Counseling that provides communication regarding the occurrence and risk of occurrence of a familial disorder is:
    a. perinatology counseling
    b. genetic counseling
    c. obstetric counseling
    d. pregnancy counseling

19. Maternal age–related chromosome abnormality risk increases after the age of:
    a. 35
    b. 32
    c. 45
    d. 40

20. Hysterosonography and hysterosonosalpingography may be frequently preferable to laparoscopy because:
    a. general anesthesia is required
    b. the ultrasound procedures are more affordable
    c. surgical complications may occur
    d. recovery time is longer

Fill-in-the-Blank

1. Cordocentesis is also known as _____.

2. An MSAFP value over _____ times the mean for a particular gestational age is suspect for _____, _____, and many other fetal abnormalities.

3. The optimal timing for a CVS is between the _____ weeks after the last menstrual period.

4. _____ is a serum protein found normally in the fetal circulatory system and produced by the fetal _____.

5. Performing amniocentesis to determine the lecithin to sphingomyelin ratio (L/S ratio) is used to determine the risk of delivering an infant with _____, usually after _____ weeks' gestation.

6. Studies suggest that _____ is the safest and most accurate of the three procedures—transcervical CVS, transabdominal CVS, and amniocentesis.

7. During amniocentesis of twins, a(an) _____ injection into the first sac/twin A after sampling ensures the second sac was entered for twin B.

8. Coelocentesis is a technique that involves the ultrasound-guided insertion of a needle into the _____ cavity through the vagina.

9. When sampling fetal blood, the anterior placenta requires _____ cordocentesis, whereas the posterior placenta allows sampling of the cord approximately _____ from the placental umbilical cord insertion.

10. Tubal catheterization is a diagnostic and _____ technique in diagnosing tubal patency via injecting and observing fluid passage into the pelvis.

11. Antibiotic prophylaxis is recommended in patients with a positive history of _____, prior to hysterosonography or hysterosonosalpingography.

12. The goal of radiotherapy is to deliver the _____ possible radiation dose to the malignant tissue and _____ the damage to the adjacent normal tissue.

13. Advantages of CVS are _____ and _____.

14. Multifetal reduction procedures have increased owing to _____-inducing drug use.

15. Indigo carmine dye is _____ in color.

16. Fetal therapy often requires access to fetal _____.

17. Fetal blood sampling occurs at the _____ cord insertion site.

18. Removal of a small amount of fluid surrounding the fetus via the maternal abdomen, for testing, is called _____.

19. Transabdominal multifetal reduction is preferred between _____ weeks gestation, and endovaginal reduction is successful between _____ weeks gestation.

20. Misdiagnosis of tubal occlusion owing to tubal spasm is a disadvantage of the _____ procedure.

Short Answer

1. Discuss reasons that pregnant women request and/or agree to amniocentesis.

2. State the ultrasound data that should be collected prior to an amniocentesis.

3. Explain how and why indigo carmine dye is used during invasive ultrasound procedures.

4. Why do recommendations suggest discarding the first small amount of amniotic fluid obtained during an amniocentesis procedure?

5. What are the advantages of hysterosonosalpingography over HSG or laparoscopy?

IMAGE EVALUATION/PATHOLOGY

Review the images and answer the following questions.

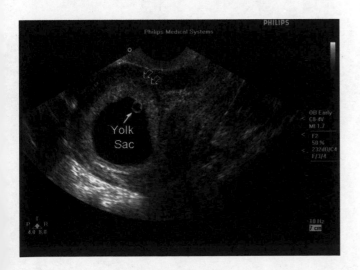

1. What type of ultrasound-guided sampling is intended for this image? See open arrows for a hint.

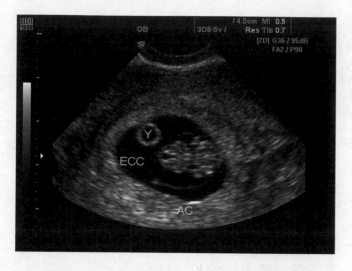

2. Name the invasive sampling procedure that this image is used for. Closely view the fetus and surroundings within the gestational sac. Name reasons this procedure is not favored over amniocentesis.

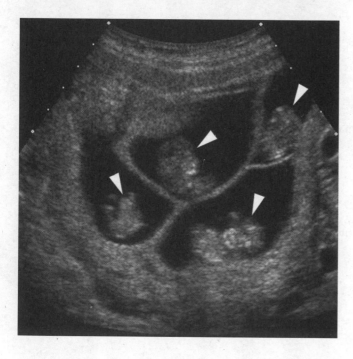

3. State the likely reason for a quadruplet pregnancy. Name the procedure that may improve the fetal survival rate for multiples.

CHAPTER 37

Assisted Reproductive Technologies

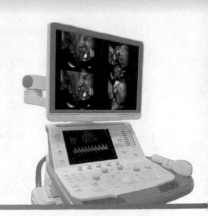

REVIEW OF GLOSSARY TERMS

Matching

Match the key terms with their definitions.

KEY TERMS

1. _____ blastocyst (embryo) transfer

2. _____ letrozole

3. _____ periovulatory period

4. _____ clomiphene citrate (CC) fertility

5. _____ in vivo fertilization

6. _____ theca lutein cysts

7. _____ cryopreservation

8. _____ infertility

9. _____ secretory phase

10. _____ estradiol

11. _____ intracytoplasmic sperm injection (ICSI)

12. _____ subfertile

13. _____ controlled ovarian hyperstimulation (COH)

14. _____ in vitro fertilization (IVF)

15. _____ proliferative phase

16. _____ assisted reproductive technologies (ARTs)

17. _____ human chorionic gonadotropin (hCG)

DEFINITIONS

a. Clinical treatments and laboratory procedures used to establish a pregnancy. This includes treatments in which both eggs and sperm are handled but in general would exclude the treatment if eggs are only stimulated and not retrieved; or if only the sperm are handled.

b. Transfer of embryo 5–6 days after egg retrieval; 4–5 days after fertilization

c. Transfer of embryo 3 days after egg retrieval, 2 days after fertilization

d. Medication used for controlled ovarian hyperstimulation of a single or multiple follicles

e. Process that promotes the development of multiple follicles in the ovary using clomiphene citrate, letrozole, or injectable gonadotropins

f. Process, usually using liquid nitrogen, to freeze embryos or gametes

g. In vitro fertilized embryo transfer into the uterine cavity at the cleavage or blastocyst stage

h. Primary hormone produced by ovarian follicles in women of childbearing age

i. Period during which the viability and survivability of both oocytes and sperm are maximum; refers to the 4- to 5-day interval ending on the day after ovulation

j. Capacity to produce offspring

k. First half of the ovarian cycle characterized by high levels of circulating follicle-stimulating hormone (FSH), which result in ovarian follicle maturation

l. An ART option rarely used, where the sperm and ova (i.e., gametes) are placed directly in the ampullary portion of the fallopian tube for in vivo fertilization

m. Hormone produced by the trophoblastic cells of the normal developing placenta or by abnormal germ cell tumors, molar pregnancies, and choriocarcinoma

18. _____ ovarian reserve

19. _____ cleavage-stage (embryo) transfer

20. _____ intrauterine insemination (IUI, aka artificial insemination)

21. _____ ovulation induction

22. _____ fertility

23. _____ menstrual phase

24. _____ fertile window

25. _____ luteal phase

26. _____ follicular phase

27. _____ hysterosalpingo contrast sonography (HyCoSy)

28. _____ gamete intrafallopian transfer (GIFT)

29. _____ ovarian hyperstimulation syndrome (OHSS)

30. _____ embryo transfer (ET)

31. _____ antral follicle count (AFC)

32. _____ fecundity

n. Fertility medication used for controlled ovarian hyperstimulation of a single or multiple follicles, used instead of clomiphene citrate

o. The ability to conceive, have ongoing pregnancy, and produce offspring

p. The number of follicles measuring 2–10 mm early in the ovarian cycle. This count helps assess a woman's potential for success with fertility treatments. It varies according to a woman's age and is used to obtain an overall sense of a woman's ovarian reserve relative to her age-matched peers.

q. Failure to achieve a pregnancy after 12 months or more of regular, unprotected intercourse, if the woman is under the age of 35 years. For those women over the age of 35 years, infertility is diagnosed if there is a failure to achieve a pregnancy after 6 months or more of regular, unprotected intercourse.

r. Injection of a single sperm into an ovum

s. Placement of seminal fluid-free sperm through the cervix directly into the uterine cavity

t. Second half of the ovarian cycle, when the corpus luteum secretes high levels of progesterone that acts on the endometrium

u. First 5 days of the menstrual cycle, characterized by endometrial shedding

v. Endovaginal sonogram which allows for the evaluation of the fallopian tubes, uterus, and ovaries by following the course of a sulfur-based dye being instilled from the cervix to the ends of the fallopian tubes. No x-ray is needed.

w. Excessive response to ovulation induction therapy, with some severe cases requiring hospitalization

x. Begins with the administration of fertility medications that induce the development of one or multiple follicles

y. Estimation of a woman's remaining follicles

z. Time just before and after mid cycle during which the endometrium may demonstrate a range of appearances spanning across both the proliferative and secretory phases

aa. Portion of the menstrual cycle during which endometrial tissue proliferates. It overlaps the menstrual phase and extends through the mid cycle.

bb. Enlarged ovaries with multiple cysts owing to abnormally high levels of hCG. Sonography plays a pivotal role in interventions designed for assisting couples struggling with infertility to successfully achieve pregnancy. This chapter covers the role of sonography in the diagnosis and treatment of infertility.

cc. Portion of the menstrual cycle characterized by an increase in circulating progesterone and during which endometrial tissue is thickest and prepared for embryo implantation

dd. Less than normal fertility though still capable of achieving pregnancy

ee. Process whereby ova and sperm come into contact *within* the body and fuse to form a zygote

ff. Process whereby ova and sperm come into contact outside the body and fuse to form a zygote from extracted ova and sperm in a laboratory setting

ANATOMY AND PHYSIOLOGY REVIEW

Image Labeling

Complete the labels in the images that follow.

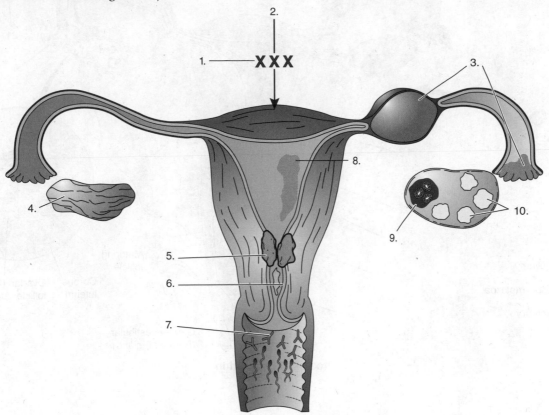

Infertility etiologies that may be overcome through ARTs

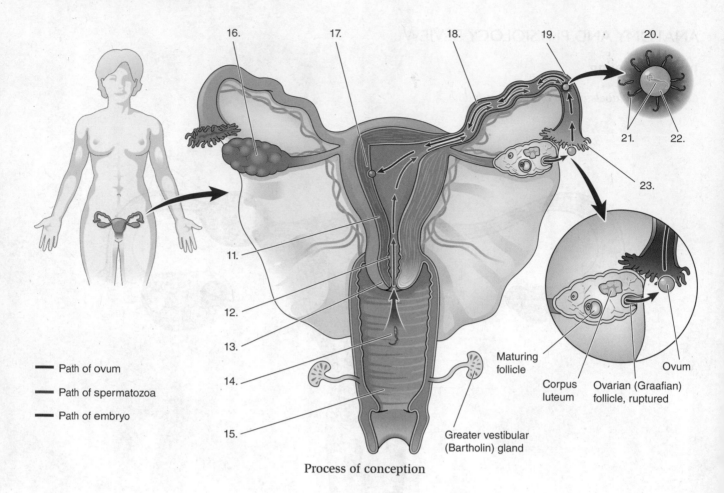

Path of ovum
Path of spermatozoa
Path of embryo

16.

17.

18.

19.

20.

21.

22.

23.

11.

12.

13.

14.

15.

Maturing
follicle

Corpus
luteum

Ovarian (Graafian)
follicle, ruptured

Ovum

Greater vestibular
(Bartholin) gland

Process of conception

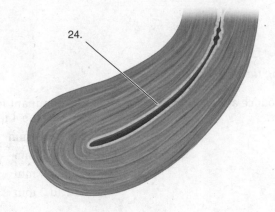

24.

A

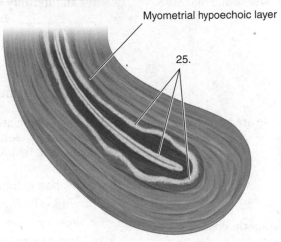

Myometrial hypoechoic layer

25.

B

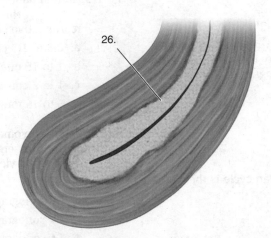

26.

C

Menstrual cycle phases

CHAPTER REVIEW

Multiple Choice

Complete each question by circling the best answer.

1. Infertility is the failure to produce a pregnancy with unprotected intercourse after:
   a. 4 months
   b. 8 months
   c. 12 months
   d. 2 years

2. Sonographic assessment of the male _____ may help to assess and diagnose infertility in a couple.
   a. scrotal anatomy
   b. epididymis
   c. vas deferens
   d. accessory glands

3. Clomiphene citrate and letrozole are known as:
   a. OI
   b. nonresponse monitoring
   c. overresponse monitoring
   d. ovulation induction agents

4. Fertilization of one egg by one sperm creates a:
   a. blastocyst
   b. gamete
   c. zygote
   d. trophoblast

5. What is the fluid-filled cavity that develops within primary follicles and is sonographically visible?
   a. Cumulus oophorus
   b. Antrum
   c. Graafian follicle
   d. Granulosa cells

6. The second half of the ovarian cycle is the:
   a. follicular phase
   b. luteal phase
   c. ovulatory phase
   d. luteum phase

7. The endometrium is thinnest during the:
   a. menstrual phase
   b. proliferative phase
   c. periovulatory phase
   d. secretory phase

8. The dominant follicle grows approximately _____ daily, in the 4 to 5 days preceding ovulation.
   a. 9 to 10 mm
   b. 6 to 7 mm
   c. 3 to 4 mm
   d. 1 to 2 mm

9. When determining the antral follicle count (AFC) for an infertility patient, only follicles between _____ are tallied.
   a. 1 and 2 cm
   b. 0.5 and 1 cm
   c. 4 and 8 mm
   d. 2 and 10 mm

10. The syndrome associated with irregularly timed menstrual cycles, elevated androgen levels often manifested by increased hair growth, hair loss, and acne is:
    a. ovarian entrapment syndrome (OES)
    b. polycystic ovary syndrome (PCOS)
    c. luteinized unruptured follicle syndrome (LUF)
    d. female reproductive syndrome (FRS)

11. Normal endometrial thickness varies from _____ through the menstrual cycle during the reproductive years.
    a. 0.5 to 1.5 cm
    b. 1 to 15 mm
    c. 1 to 2 cm
    d. 3 to 16 mm

12. Polyps, myomas, synechiae, retained products of conception, endometrial hyperplasia, and carcinoma can best be viewed using:
    a. SIS
    b. EV sonography
    c. TV sonography
    d. TA sonography

13. Distortion of the uterine cavity, interference of uterine/endometrial blood flow, and tubal ostia occlusion are mostly related to:
    a. an abnormal septum
    b. mucus collection
    c. submucosal fibroids
    d. adenomyosis

14. The preferred imaging method to ensure fallopian tube patency is:
    a. MRI
    b. SIS
    c. laparoscopy
    d. HSG

15. The prevailing reason for male infertility is:
    a. varicoceles
    b. testicular failure
    c. idiopathic causes
    d. vasoepididymal obstruction

16. A baseline scan is performed:
    a. following IVF-ET
    b. within the first few days of menstrual flow
    c. 3 weeks post IVF-ET
    d. at the end of menstrual flow

17. Intracytoplasmic sperm injection (ICSI) is:
    a. the injection of one sperm into the cytoplasm of one egg
    b. in vivo method of inseminating a single ovum via the fallopian tube
    c. a technique that treats immobile sperm intratesticular to increase progressive motility
    d. extraction of ova cytoplasm followed by sperm injection and replacement

18. For many etiologies of infertility, the first step in treatment is:
    a. baseline sonography
    b. COH
    c. OI
    d. OHSS

19. In an embryo transfer procedure, the embryo along with its surrounding culture media
    a. is not visualized until 5 weeks, 5 days
    b. appears anechoic (black) once released from the catheter
    c. appears echogenic (bright white) once released from the catheter
    d. is seen within the catheter tip

20. The stage of an embryo at 2 or 3 days after fertilization is known as:
    a. gamete
    b. zygote
    c. blastocyst
    d. cleavage

21. An embryologist uses a container responsible for moving embryos into the uterine cavity. The container is a:
    a. speculum
    b. TV biopsy guide
    c. indwelling catheter
    d. transfer catheter

22. EV sonography is utilized to detect a gestational sac:
    a. by 5 weeks after a woman's last menstrual period
    b. at 6.5 weeks from LMP
    c. 2.5 weeks after egg retrieval/fertilization
    d. post LMP 4 weeks

Fill-in-the-Blank

1. Most fertility centers will follow patients through their first trimester with the first sonogram often being scheduled at approximately _____ weeks EGA.

2. Serious complications of ovarian stimulation techniques used in assisted reproduction are _____ and _____.

3. _____ is frequently linked with timed intercourse, intrauterine insemination (IUI), or in vitro fertilization-embryo transfer (IVF-ET).

4. The normal ovarian/menstrual cycle lasts _____ days, beginning on the first day of a woman's menses, and extending to the _____ day of her next menses.

5. Day 14 of the menstrual cycle is usually when _____ occurs.

6. The corpus luteum begins to degenerate about _____ days after ovulation if fertilization does not occur.

7. A surge in _____ causes the dominant follicle to rupture, at which time the _____ will erupt from the ovary.

8. The mean diameter of a dominant follicle, at the time of ovulation, is _____ mm.

9. _____ acquisition can provide automated counting of follicles.

10. A "string of pearls" is associated with _____ and increased ovarian surface area.

11. The endometrium consists of a _____ layer and a _____ layer.

12. IUI is _____.

13. A cause of female infertility known for uterine scarring and usually related to pregnancy loss showing absence or discontinuation of endometrial stripe is _____.

14. Sonography of the endometrium is able to assess _____, _____ flow, _____ movements, presence of intracavitary lesions, and the presence of intracavitary fluid.

15. Adenomyosis is the presence of endometrial tissue within the _____.

16. Semen analysis includes sperm _____, _____, and _____.

17. The classic appearance of multiple tubular veins superior to the testes which can contribute to infertility is described as _____.

18. Once follicles are considered to be mature, _____ or _____ is administered to induce ovulation.

19. An endometrial thickness of less than _____ millimeters (mm) is useful in predicting poor implantation rates in in vitro fertilization cycles.

20. Varicocele is determined by _____ or more veins measuring _____ mm or greater with or without the Valsalva technique.

Short Answer

1. A female fertility patient presents for ovarian reserve assessment. Explain what she should expect.

2. Discuss the EV appearance of the normal uterine endometrium during the three phases of the menstrual cycle.

3. A couple who has been infertile for 2 years is seeking medical help. Testing has determined the sperm concentration to be slightly low. Explain the most likely and probably least costly process to assist with their infertility.

IMAGE EVALUATION/PATHOLOGY

Review the images and answer the following questions.

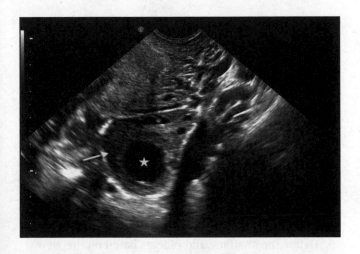

1. What imaging method was used to collect this image? Identify the image depicted by the arrow and anatomy with a star. Is blood flow documented?

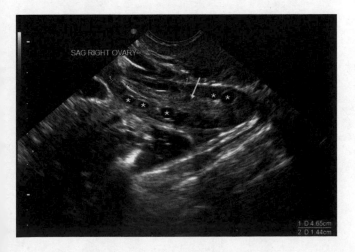

2. State the anatomy, laterality, and view of this image. What are the structure dimensions?
State what the stars and arrow are identifying.

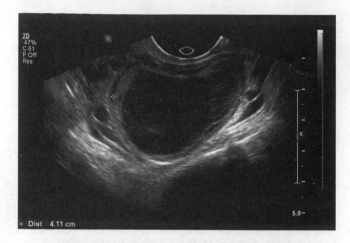

3. Explain the image.

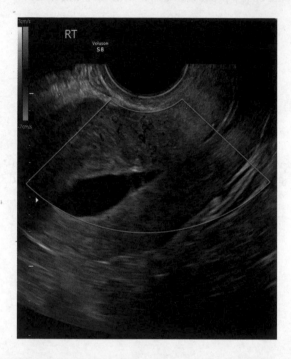

4. Explain the image and the anomaly.

5. Define the anatomy and process based on the view of the endometrium.

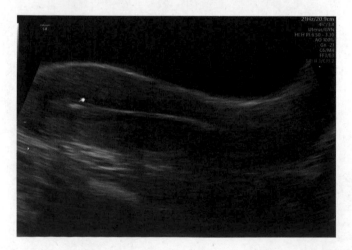

CHAPTER 38

Complementary Imaging of the Female Reproductive System

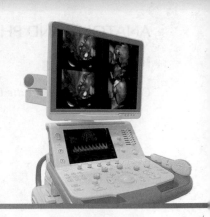

REVIEW OF GLOSSARY TERMS

Matching

Match the key terms with their definitions.

KEY TERMS

1. _____ high signal intensity

2. _____ time to repetition (TR)

3. _____ hypointense

4. _____ sequence(s)

5. _____ graded-compression technique

6. _____ hyperintense

7. _____ fat saturation (FS)

8. _____ isointense

9. _____ gadolinium

10. _____ MRI weightings (weighted image)

11. _____ hybrid imaging

12. _____ time to echo (TE)

13. _____ spectroscopic

DEFINITIONS

a. Commonly used MRI contrast agent
b. Utilizing mixed imaging parameters (T2 and T1) to create an optimal image
c. Having an intensity greater than surrounding structures
d. Set of parameters used to create a specific type of image (T1, T2, T2 FS)
e. Time between the application of the 90-degree pulse and the peak of the echo signal
f. Commonly used MRI technique to suppress signal from fat tissue
g. Method to detect, determine, and quantify the molecular component of tissue
h. Time between pulses in a series of pulses for a single image
i. Applying pressure (compression) to displace structures such as bowel to bring intra-abdominal structures within the focal zone
j. Having an intensity less than surrounding structures
k. Having the same image intensity as surrounding structures
l. Arrangement of radio frequency pulses and gradients that combine to create an image
m. Signal that depicts brightness on the MRI image

ANATOMY AND PHYSIOLOGY REVIEW

Image Labeling

Complete the labels in the images that follow.

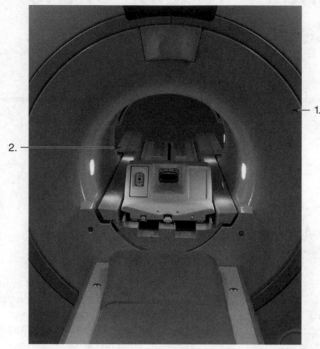

Identify structures the arrows point toward.

MRI unit

CHAPTER REVIEW

Multiple Choice

Complete each question by circling the best answer.

1. Choose the imaging modality with the largest field of view.
   a. MRI
   b. CT
   c. US
   d. Both MRI and CT

2. MRI is based on the ability to excite _____ protons.
   a. cation
   b. hydrogen
   c. negative
   d. chromium

3. Name the device responsible for transmitting radiofrequency within the MRI unit.
   a. NMV
   b. Gradient coil
   c. Antenna
   d. Magnetic field

4. T2 and T1 are types of MRI:
   a. weighting
   b. images
   c. values
   d. displays

5. The MRI technique to selectively remove the signal from adipose protons is:
   a. TE
   b. TR
   c. FS
   d. NMV

6. Recent research has shown that gadolinium can accumulate in the human:
   a. liver
   b. spleen
   c. brain
   d. pancreas

7. CT attenuation is the _____ of intensity as the radiation passes through a patient.
   a. gradual loss
   b. gradual increase
   c. coefficient
   d. value

8. What are the measurement units, from white to black, that CT uses to display images?
   a. Duplex
   b. Range
   c. Monochrome
   d. Hounsfield

9. Select the modality that offers the best tissue differentiation.
   a. US
   b. CT
   c. MRI
   d. CT and MRI

10. Vaginal agenesis can be responsible for:
    a. septa
    b. hematometrocolpos
    c. Gartner duct cysts
    d. a homogeneous MRI image

11. A malignant multilocular cervical cyst is known as:
    a. adenoma malignum
    b. cervicitis
    c. tunnel cluster
    d. endocervical hyperplasia

12. Name the imaging modality initially used to locate uterine fibroids.
    a. US
    b. CT
    c. MRI
    d. CT and MRI

13. _____ is used most often to predict the response of fibroids to uterine artery embolization.
    a. US
    b. CT
    c. MRI
    d. CT and MRI

14. MRI adds extensive diagnostic data to uterine studies by displaying how many uterine distinct soft tissue zones?
    a. Two
    b. Three
    c. Four
    d. Five

15. MRI T2 imaging displays simple ovarian cysts and simple paraovarian cysts as:
    a. high signal
    b. intermediate signal
    c. low signal
    d. fat saturation signal

16. Select an advantage that CT imaging has over MRI imaging as a complementary modality to ultrasound.
    a. No radiation exposure
    b. Faster image acquisition
    c. Extensive multiplanar positioning
    d. Superior tissue differentiation

17. Dehiscence is seen:
    a. within the fundal endometrium
    b. within the fundal myometrium
    c. at the level of the external os
    d. in the lower uterine segment

18. The two most likely modalities to demonstrate cervical competence are:
    a. CT, MRI
    b. CT, US
    c. US, MRI
    d. MRI, CT

19. Graded compression is a(n) _____ technique that is helpful in locating the:
    a. US, appendix
    b. CT, fallopian tubes
    c. CT, adnexal fibroids
    d. MRI, pelvic hernia

20. Choose the reason uterine müllerian duct errors are imaged with MRI.
    a. It displays related anomalies such as kidney and vertebral body involvement.
    b. Its strength in evaluating soft tissue uterine configurations
    c. Its ability to image the difficult body habitus
    d. The cost factor

Fill-in-the-blank

1. _____ is the most sensitive diagnostic imaging test for uterine fibroids.

2. A group of parameters used to create a specific type of image is known as MRI _____.

3. _____ is a method to detect, determine, and quantify the molecular component of tissue.

4. MRI imaging relies on the ability to excite _____ protons contained in water within the body tissues.

5. MRI contrast administration of _____ during pregnancy is controversial.

6. CT imaging risks decrease into the _____ and _____ trimesters; however, research has shown that a slightly increased risk of childhood cancer is associated with radiation in utero.

7. The cost of an MRI examination is _____ compared to CT and US.

8. Appendicitis on MRI shows an appendiceal diameter over _____ mm, wall thickness over _____ mm, high signal intensity contents on T2 weighted images, and surrounding _____.

9. MRI cannot visualize non-hydrogen structures in the pelvis such as _____ or _____ devices.

10. T2 demonstrates _____ amniotic fluid filling the incompetent, dilated cervical canal up to the level of the "closed" cervix.

11. Incomplete _____ of the endometrium and myometrium with an intact serosal layer characterizes uterine dehiscence.

12. The diagnosis of cystic teratoma is reasonably unequivocal because of the fat within the mass, which MRI detects with specific _____ sequences.

13. MRI diagnosis of endometrioma is based on the detection of _____ products of different ages within a unilateral or bilateral adnexal mass.

14. Fallopian tube fibroids are best characterized with MRI because this complementary modality can define the _____ location due to its exceptional tissue differentiation ability.

15. Poorly defined polyps and _____ masses may not be distinguishable with US, whereas MRI is usually able to differentiate these anomalies.

16. An advantage of MRI as compared to US of the uterine myometrium and endometrium is MRI's ability to depict defined _____.

17. When hyperplasia is suspected, MRI may only offer an advantage over US when the _____ approach is not available or when the endometrial images demonstrate dubious findings.

18. During pregnancy, the _____ is poorly visualized as the signal is augmented and approaches the signal of the outer myometrium. The layers are seen again _____ days after delivery.

19. The modalities, _____ and _____, are capable of viewing anatomy in many planes, which includes orthogonal and oblique.

20. Both _____ and _____ are widely utilized for cancer staging.

Short Answer

1. Compare US, MRI, and CT imaging of the uterine endometrium.

2. Consider US and MRI in the pregnant female when appendicitis is suspected.

IMAGE EVALUATION/PATHOLOGY

Review the images and answer the following questions.

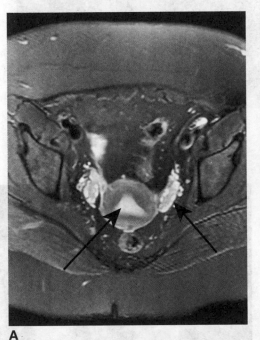 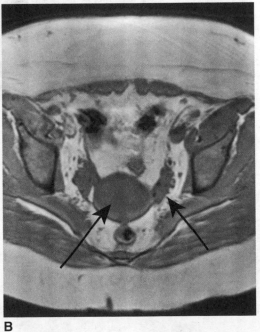

A   B

1. Is image A T2 or T1? Is image B T2 or T1? What structure is the left arrow pointing toward in both images? What structure is the right arrow pointing toward in both images?

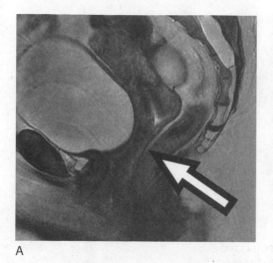

A

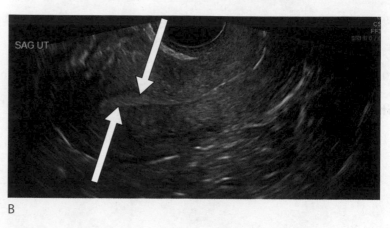

B

2. Name the structure the arrows are directed toward in both images.

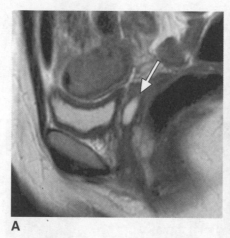

A

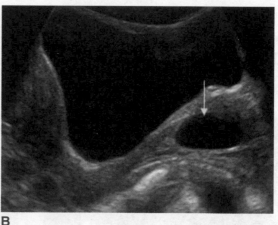

B

3. What is the arrow directed to in images A and B?

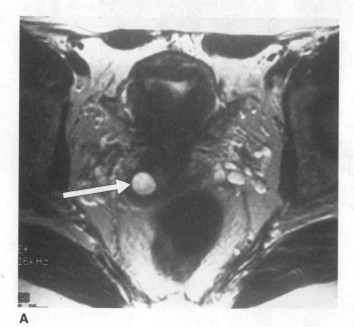

A

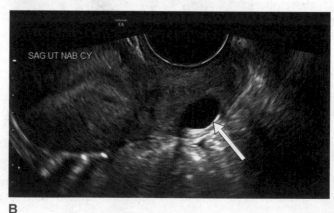

B

4. What is the structure the arrow points toward in images A and B?

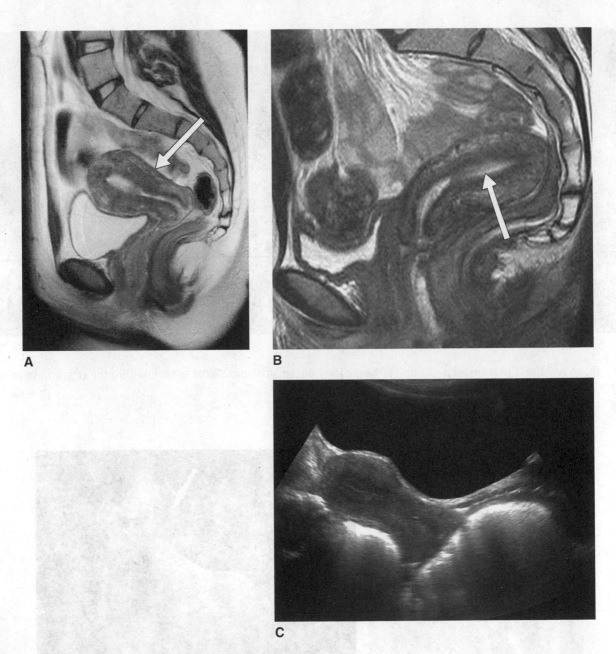

A

B

C

5. Name the uterine position for images A, B, and C. What is the anatomic region depicted by the arrows in images A and B?

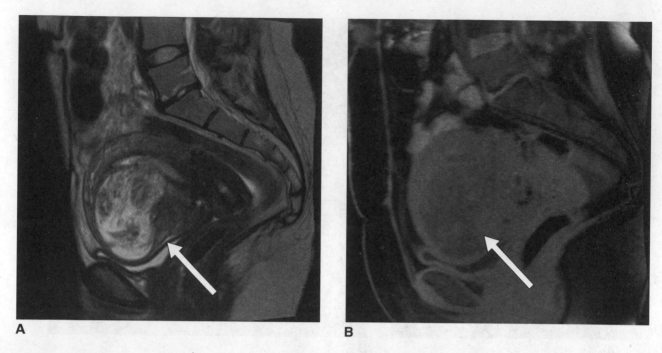

6. Is image A T2 or T1? Is image B T2 or T1? Name the imaged structure. What is seen within the organ in both images (*arrow*)?

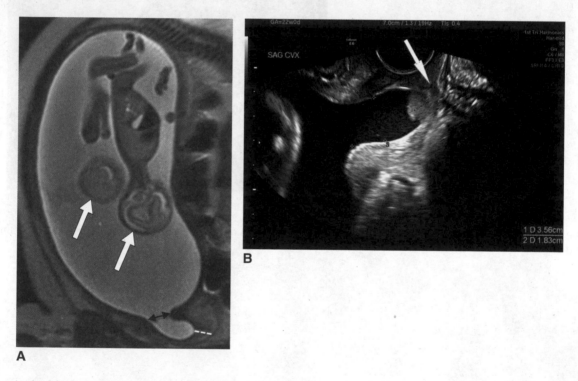

7. What is the black double arrow line directed at in image A? Name the MRI weighting used to acquire this image. Explain what the white arrow shows in image B.

CHAPTER 39

3D and 4D Imaging in Obstetrics and Gynecology

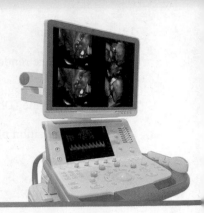

REVIEW OF GLOSSARY TERMS

Matching

Match the key terms with their definitions.

KEY TERMS

1. _____ 4D imaging

2. _____ spatiotemporal image correlation (STIC)

3. _____ region of interest (ROI)

4. _____ C-plane

5. _____ transparency

6. _____ 3D ultrasound

7. _____ orthogonal planes

8. _____ voxel

9. _____ sweep

10. _____ volume ultrasound

11. _____ volume of interest (aka render box)

12. _____ reference dot

13. _____ 3D volume or volume data set

14. _____ threshold

15. _____ pixel

16. _____ maximum

17. _____ multiplanar reconstruction (MPR)

18. _____ tomographic ultrasound imaging (aka multislice)

DEFINITIONS

a. Display algorithm for viewing more than one plane simultaneously; frequently sagittal, transverse, and coronal planes that are 90 degrees to each other, also known as sectional planes or orthogonal planes

b. Smallest unit of a 3D volume, consisting of a length, width, and depth

c. Imaging technology involving the automatic or manual acquisition and display of a series of 2D images

d. Rotates the MPR or volume rendering horizontally. The letter "X" flipping over top to bottom, repeatedly

e. Rotates the MPR or volume rendering vertically, spinning right to left in a circular pattern on its stem

f. The MPR placed 90 degrees to the acquisition plane; synonymous to the Y-plane; shows the volume acquisition angle

g. Collection of acquired 2D images

h. The smallest unit of a 2D image, has height and length

i. Planes that are always at right angles (90 degrees) to each other; typically sagittal, transverse, and coronal

j. Rolls the MPR or volume rendering clockwise or counterclockwise; rotates around a central point (i.e., car or bicycle wheel, analog clock)

k. Point where all three orthogonal planes intersect within the volume; depicts the same anatomic point in three orthogonal planes; also called the marker dot

l. Standard file format for handling, storing, printing, and transmitting information in any form of medical imaging (i.e., radiology, pathology, laboratory, etc.)

m. Area of data acquisition for the 3D/4D volume

n. Determines whether the voxels will be more or less see-through

o. 3D rendering mode that displays the surface or skin of the body without displaying the underlying anatomy

19. _____ B-plane

20. _____ surface rendering

21. _____ digital imaging and communication in medicine (DICOM)

22. _____ acquisition plane

23. _____ A-plane

24. _____ look line

25. _____ minimum mode

26. _____ philtrum

27. _____ Z-axis

28. _____ temporal

29. _____ Y-axis

30. _____ X-axis

31. _____ spatial

p. Technique used to acquire and display a volume data set of the fetal heart; the volume displays as a 4D cine sequence of the beating heart
q. Filter used to eliminate low-level echoes
r. Display format in which the data are viewed as a series of parallel tomographic images similar to the display methods traditionally used in computed tomography and magnetic resonance imaging
s. Relating to distance or position
t. Defines information contained within the volume rendering
u. Continuously updated display of volume information; also known as real-time 3D ultrasound and live 3D ultrasound
v. Coronal plane 90 degrees to the A-plane and transmit beam; 2D imaging does not allow imaging on this reconstructed; synonymous to the Z-plane
w. The median cleft between the nose and upper lip
x. An adjustable line indicating the plane depth of a structure that we manually select to view desired anatomy (superior myometrium, endometrium, posterior myometrium). The graphic indicating the direction we view the MPR or volume rendering
y. Method to remove echoes from fluid-filled structures rending them black on the MPR
z. The distance the transducer moves during acquisition
aa. Relating to time
bb. The acquisition plane of the multiplanar reconstruction display (MPR); synonymous to the X-plane
cc. Reduction or elimination of weak, soft-tissue echoes to highlight bony structures
dd. Term used to describe both 3D and 4D imaging
ee. The plane for the acquired data set, usually the A-plane MPR

ANATOMY AND PHYSIOLOGY REVIEW

Image Labeling

Complete the labels in the images that follow.

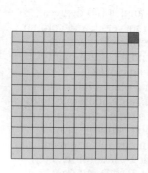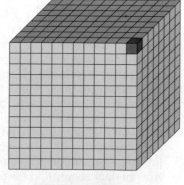

PIXEL = 2D **VOXEL = 3D**

1. Name smallest unit of 2D.

2. Name smallest unit of 3D.

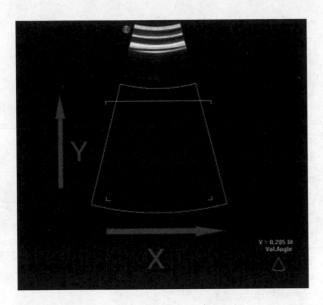

4-6. Name orthogonal planes from left to right.

3. Name planes of the ROI box.

CHAPTER REVIEW

Multiple Choice

Complete each question by circling the best answer.

1. 3D/4D imaging uses reconstruction abilities similar to:
   a. nuclear medicine
   b. angiography
   c. computed tomography
   d. digital mammography

2. Pixel is defined as:
   a. picture element
   b. cube acquisition
   c. data set
   d. planes Y and Z

3. 2D transducers require _____ acquisition to produce 3D images.
   a. automated
   b. concentric
   c. freehand
   d. annular

4. The ability to "see through" the voxel depends on the:
   a. resolution setting
   b. gain setting
   c. mode setting
   d. transparency setting

5. Evaluation of hypoechoic structures is enhanced with the adjustment of the:
   a. maximum and skeletal modes
   b. minimum and inversion modes
   c. surface-rendering mode
   d. X, Y, and Z planes

6. Anomalies of the fetal heart are best detected using _____ technology.
   a. VOCAL
   b. scalpel
   c. glass body
   d. STIC

7. All of the following are clinical applications for 3D/4D gynecologic ultrasound except:
   a. congenital uterine anomalies
   b. fetal lip characteristics
   c. IUD location
   d. infertility evaluation

8. Select the view required to display diagnostic fetal heart images utilizing STIC technology.
   a. Coronal AP heart
   b. Decubitus heart displaying LVOT
   c. Apical four chamber
   d. PA four chamber

9. Uterine volume imaging displays all except:
   a. Essure™ device
   b. IUD arm position
   c. bicornuate IUP
   d. urinary incontinence

10. What is not a common clinical application for a 3D/4D obstetric imaging?
    a. Nasal bone interrogation
    b. STIC
    c. Adnexal assessment
    d. Extremity evaluation

11. Limitations of 3D/4D imaging are all except:
    a. poor 2D acquisition reveals subpar 3D imaging
    b. surface-rendering ability
    c. fetal movement
    d. low amniotic fluid

12. A reference dot is:
    a. also known as a look dot
    b. the point where two planes intersect within the volume
    c. measured by distance or position
    d. the point where three orthogonal planes intersect within the volume

13. In 3D imaging, a filter used to eliminate low-level echoes is called:
    a. threshold
    b. scalpel
    c. transparency
    d. minimum

14. The 3D mode that views hypoechoic structures and displays them as a solid structure or creates a digital cast of the object is:
    a. render mode
    b. texture mode
    c. inversion mode
    d. light mode

15. The rendering mode, glass body, or transparency is used with:
    a. basic slicing
    b. color Doppler
    c. casting
    d. orthogonal plane manipulation

16. Planes that are positioned 90 degrees to each other in 3D imaging are called:
    a. reference planes
    b. multiplanes
    c. orthogonal planes
    d. tomographic planes

17. The rendering mode useful for evaluating the spine, extremities, and cranial sutures is:
    a. medium mode
    b. minimum mode
    c. skeletal mode
    d. multiplanar

18. The smallest unit of a 3D data set is:
    a. picture element
    b. voxel
    c. sensor
    d. X plane

19. Distortion of anatomy can be caused by:
    a. reference dot position
    b. shadowing
    c. narrow fan sweeps
    d. movement of anatomy

20. The central dot seen in the MPR views shows the intersection of the planes and the _____ location.
    a. pivot
    b. volume orientation
    c. surface rendering
    d. sweep

Fill-in-the-Blank

1. The term used to describe both 3D and 4D imaging is _____ imaging.

2. _____ ultrasound provides anatomical views that are difficult or even impossible to obtain with 2D ultrasound.

3. When a sagittal uterus is imaged with 3D, the B-plane displays a _____ uterus and the C-plane image displays a _____ uterus.

4. The _____ box determines the amount of information displayed in the A and B planes, whereas the determination of the amount of information in the C-plane is through the size of the _____ angle.

5. _____ transducers obtain conventional 2D images as well as 3D images.

6. A real-time volume acquisition of the fetal heart is performed with _____ correlation.

7. The _____ plane, adjustable before or after the acquisition, removes data between the line graphic and the transducer, allowing for editing of the volume.

8. 3D rendering mode that displays the surface or skin of the body without displaying the underlying anatomy is _____.

9. A _____ image of anatomy cannot be obtained with conventional 2D imaging.

10. Planes that are always at right angles (90 degrees) to each other; typically sagittal, transverse, and coronal are known as _____ planes.

11. Conventional 2D imaging does not display a _____ view.

12. Tomographic ultrasound imaging is also known as _____ imaging.

13. Pelvic floor imaging that includes both grayscale and volume images requires the use of a _____.

14. 3D is referred to as static imaging whereas 4D is called _____ or _____ imaging.

15. The internal _____ in 3D/4D transducers provide spatial information, allowing for precise volume reconstruction.

16. Acquisition _____, a user-controlled parameter, changes the quality of the resulting data set.

17. Evaluation of bony structures is best with _____, _____, or _____ mode, whereas surface-rendering mode brings out the _____ line.

18. _____, used in conjunction with color Doppler modes, highlights vascular anatomy by increasing the transparency of the overlying tissue.

19. _____ volume acquisition techniques allow the use of conventional 2D transducers. In this method, examiners manually sweep or move the transducer through the area of interest.

20. Regarding 4D ultrasound, the _____ the volume rate, the closer to real time the images appear.

Short Answer

1. List common artifacts seen with 3D imaging due to fetal movement during image acquisition.

2. Explain the benefit of obtaining data sets.

3. State common clinical applications of 3D/4D in gynecology.

IMAGE EVALUATION/PATHOLOGY

Review the images and answer the following questions.

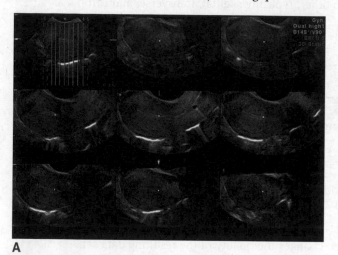

A

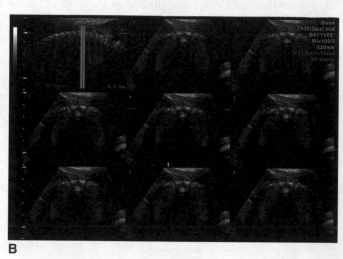

B

1. Name the type of imaging seen in the image. Explain how the upper left image relates to the entire study.

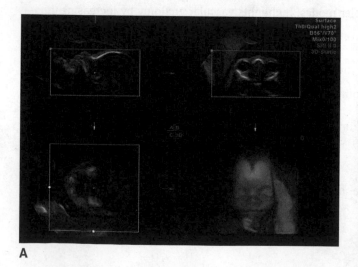

A

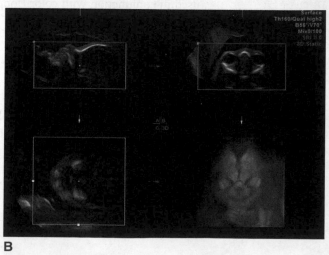

B

2. Explain image A. Compare and contrast it with image B. Discuss the reason for the image difference.